Kari's Destiny

~ No More Tomorrows

by

Olivia Claire High

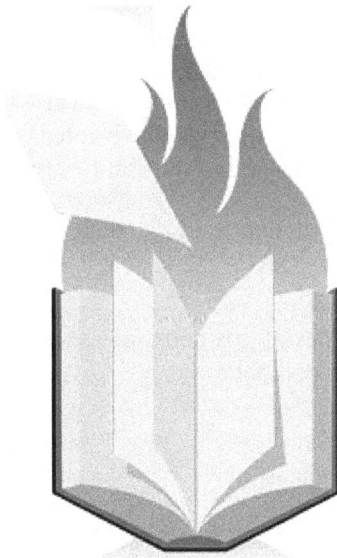

Fireside Publications
Oxford, Florida 34484

Fireside Publications
5144 Harbour Drive
Oxford, Florida 34484

www.firesidepubs.com

Printed in the United States of America

This book is not a work of fiction. Rather, it is a true story of one family's tragic life-journey. A few names may have been changed or omitted to protect privacy of people not directly related to the family. Otherwise, people, businesses, events and incidences are accurate to the best of the author's knowledge. All pictures are used with the consent of the persons who are the subject of the photo.

For additional copies of this book, please visit:
www.firesidepubs.com,   or

Contact the author at:
Joeclaire2424@comcast.net

Dedication

To all those who are suffering from leukemia and to the victims who lost their battle against the disease; and to the families who suffer along with their loved ones.

To my granddaughter, Kari Elizabeth Moseley, who reminds me every day what it means to have true courage.

To my late mother, Elizabeth Brown who was there all through my daughter's illness offering me strength and support when I needed it the most.

Acknowledgements

Love and many thanks to my husband, Joe for his help and encouragement.

All my love to my family who fill my heart with happiness.

My appreciation to Lois Bennett for publishing my daughter's story, so others could have the opportunity to know about my special little girl, Kari Suzanne.

And to God, who is with me always.

Prologue

My first daughter, Kathleen Marie was born in June, 1958. My husband, Joe, and I nicknamed her Kathy. She was born with wispy blonde hair, light colored eyes, and a cleft lip. I didn't get to see her until the day I brought her home from the hospital because the nurses didn't want to upset me. I guess they thought since I was only eighteen they needed to protect me from the shock. I was so naïve it didn't occur to me to insist I wanted to see my baby.

A friend who had just given birth to a boy with Down's syndrome a couple of months earlier came to visit me in the hospital. She told me to be thankful my baby's problem could be fixed. By the time I finally did get to hold Kathy I didn't think she looked that bad.

But it did upset me later when I took her out in public, and some people stared at her or made rude remarks. My doctor said it was natural for me to feel embarrassed by Kathy's appearance. I felt offended by his preconceived assumption that I was ashamed of her. No one wants to be told they have an ugly child.

Kathy had surgery when she was nine weeks old. It was so successful that people rarely noticed the thin little scar on her lip. She didn't ask about it until she was five years old. When she wanted to know what happened, I explained that her lip didn't grow together and the doctor fixed it. She thought the scar was special enough to share for show and tell in kindergarten.

My second child was born in October, 1960. Autumn is my favorite season of the year. I love the crisp air and the fresh scent of rain that washes away the last of the summer dust and heat. I think it's one of nature's many marvelous phenomena the way the trees gradually change their leaves into all the different brilliant colors of fall. Sometimes I can't resist picking them up and even keeping them for a while.

As soon as Joe came home from his high school teaching job that day, I told him I was having strong cramping. Since the baby was due the next day, it seemed logical that this was significant enough to alert the doctor. He examined me and told Joe to take me for a walk near the hospital to keep things going. We strolled along until I started having quite a bit of pressure in my back and decided we shouldn't delay any longer.

I sympathize with women who endure the gripping pains of a long, difficult labor, straining to bring their children into the world. I was fortunate not to have to go through too much of that. I don't know if the Lamaze method was around then, but I figured out on my own if I tried to relax when each contraction started, the pain wasn't too bad.

I didn't have a long labor with Kathy; and this time things were progressing much faster than anyone expected. Two nurses helped me onto a gurney and took me down the hallway toward the delivery room. I heard one of them say in an undertone that my doctor hadn't arrived because someone called the wrong one. The other nurse told her to be quiet because she might frighten me. I was busy thinking I hoped someone was going to be there to help because a little head had just popped out between my legs!

My doctor's office was across the street from the hospital, and he did arrive in time to assist with the delivery. Fifty minutes after I entered the hospital I was told I had another baby girl and she was fine. Joe and I named our new daughter Kari Suzanne.

Later that night as I cuddled this new little life in my arms I felt the joy of being able to hold her so soon after her birth, since that privilege had been denied me with Kathy. I just couldn't seem to look at Kari enough. I gently pressed a finger into her tiny palm and watched in fascination as her little hand slowly closed over it. Such a simple response, but I felt a huge rush of love at that first trusting touch.

I examined her face, still wrinkled and slightly pink from her months immersed within her watery domain. Her facial contortions made me smile as I unfolded the tip of one ear that was slightly bent. Her ears seemed a little too big for her narrow face, but I thought she looked wonderful. I held her close and stroked her soft cheek. I felt so happy I almost couldn't breathe for a moment. A sense of peace came over me as though I was being surrounded by a lovely violin melody that flows through you until you can't tell the difference between the music and the rhythm of your heart.

We're all born with the potential to become ill or have a serious accident, and of course we all face eventual death. But I'm sure no one would be thinking about that when they'd just given birth to a healthy baby. I certainly didn't. I had no indication of the anguish that was to come. I saw only what was evident to me and felt the joy that was appropriate to the occasion.

This story is about what fate had in store for my second daughter and how that destiny affected my life and the lives of those closest to me.

In Memory of:
Kari Suzanne High
We will always miss you.

No More Tomorrows
No more Sadness
No more Pain

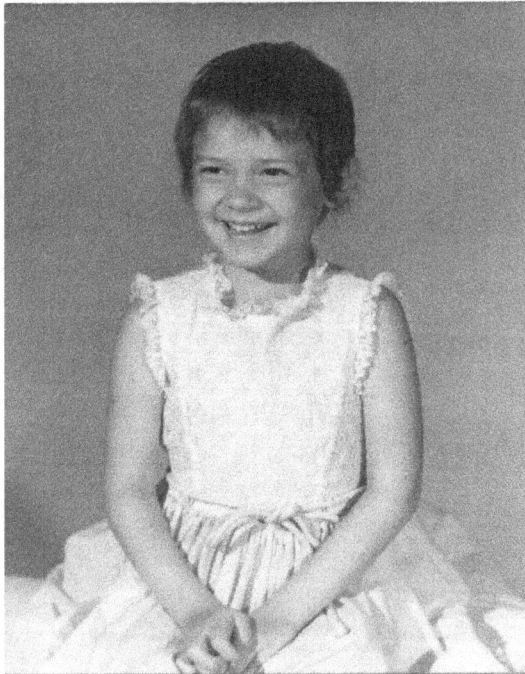

October 14, 1960 – September 15, 1966

Photo Date: June 1966 ~ 3 months prior to Kari's passing.

4

Chapter One

Kari and I left the hospital two days later under a clear, blue sky. Leaves swirled gently in the air, fluttering gracefully to the ground in scattered piles of color. My parents resided in Napa, California a couple hours away from where I lived in the smaller town of Oroville. My mother planned to stay with us for a few days. Kari lay swaddled in a white blanket that was a perfect background for her dark hair. I peeked at her as she slept secure in her own private world.

I inhaled the fresh October air, as the nurse pushed me in a wheelchair to where my family stood eagerly waiting to greet their newest member. Kathy clutched the new doll Joe and I had given her. She had her baby and I had mine.

Like Kathy, Kari was an easy baby to care for. She progressed at her own pace as children do. She subtly tossed out her own distinctive little net easily capturing us within her delicate snare. We were drawn to her sweetness like bears to a honey pot.

I love babies. They come from their special cloistered world with their own unique chemistry. They have a certain mystery about them that intrigues me. I can't help wondering what goes on inside their pure little minds, especially when I see the myriad of expressions flitting across their face. Their needs are pretty elemental and unsophisticated; feed me, clothe me, shelter me, love me.

I wanted to do the very best I could for my children, so their lives would turn out to be as happy as possible. Our environment, our genes, and our decisions all influence us, but the inevitability of our fate will have the final say.

I think the greatest rabbit we could pull out of the magic hat of life would be to figure out a way to alter an especially bad destiny. Maybe some people do manage such a feat, but if you can't, you're left to deal with whatever comes your way. Even a very clever person can't write the entire script for their life.

I was finally old enough to vote in my first presidential election in 1960. My Aunt June, who lived in Oroville was Kari's godmother. She thought Kari looked like President Kennedy's son, born that same year. I'm not sure if that was a compliment since he was a boy, but he sure was a cute little guy. It did strike me at the time how different their lives were. One was the son of a president and the other a school teacher's daughter. It wouldn't matter to them in their infancy because they were too young to care about that kind of thing.

And certainly no one could possibly know how significant the year 1963 would end up being for those two children.

Kari gave us a health scare early in December 1960. I'd taken her to the doctor the day before because she had a cold. He prescribed nose drops to help her breathe easier. She was very lethargic the next day and would only take a little formula from her bottle.

When Joe got home late that afternoon he thought she looked unnaturally pale. I called our doctor and he notified a pediatrician who had to come from the nearby city of Chico. We were told to take Kari to our local hospital, and the doctor would meet us.

I'd just left there less than two months earlier filled with happiness; and now I was returning under a cloud of uncertainty. I felt like Joe and I were playing a strange game of tennis, except that this wasn't a game. It began with Kathy being born with her cleft lip and then having the ball back in our court when she had her surgery. Now the ball was out of our court again. Would we be able to get it back?

I felt a wrenching ache when I had to hand Kari over to a nurse and watch her disappear down a hallway with my baby. Joe and I sat and waited for what we hoped wouldn't be bad news. Darkness had fallen outside. The room's ceiling lights cast a harsh glare over the pale walls, surrounding us with a garish glow. Each minute that ticked by tore away at my confidence.

Joe and I jerked out of our chairs in our anxiousness to hear the results of the pediatrician's examination when he finally came to see us. He explained that Kari had a subnormal temperature besides her extreme pallor and listlessness. He initially thought she might have been suffering from mcningitis. Although he ruled that possibility out, he wasn't able to give us a conclusive diagnosis, except to say that perhaps she'd had a reaction to the nose drops.

I thought we would be bringing Kari home then, but the doctor told us he wanted to keep her in the hospital as a precaution. So once again Joe and I were forced to entrust one of our babies to the care of a medical staff just like we had to do when Kathy had her surgery.

We walked toward the exit and opened the door to a heavy rain. I barely noticed the chilly drops splashing against my face as we made our way between two enormous palm trees. They stood like a couple of gigantic sentinels with their massive long fingered fronds dripping water onto the sodden grass. We walked through the shadowy opening in the wrought iron fence with its fleur-de-lis design pointing upward like clusters of miniature spears.

The car's chilly interior greeted us with a damp cold. I took one last look over my shoulder at the row of hospital windows wondering which room Kari might be in. Joe drove us home through the silent, empty streets. I wore a warm jacket, but I couldn't stop shivering.

Questions started to pop up inside my head. Would Kari be okay? How long would she have to stay in the hospital? What was the matter with her? Was it just the nose drops, as the doctor said, or was something more serious going to come from this?

I felt like a key player in a drama who didn't know her lines. I clasped my cold hands in my lap. I hated the feeling of helplessness. My baby was ill. If only I could do something besides sitting and fretting. Then I did the only thing I could think of. I asked God for His assistance.

The idea came to me that perhaps He would help if I showed Him I was willing to give something in return. I silently vowed to start attending church on a regular basis again if the Almighty would let my baby be well. I didn't think of my request as trying to strike a bargain, but rather I considered it an honest pledge to do my part.

The phone rang the next morning with the wonderful news that Kari was fine and the doctor had signed the release for her to go home. I was finally able to relax and let go of the tension that had gripped my body for the last several hours. I realized Joe and I had come through another crisis involving one of our children. I offered up several heartfelt prayers thanking God, as I drove to the hospital.

Some of the nurses were waiting to greet me when I arrived. One of them held Kari while the others gathered around her chattering that silly kind of prattle we all tend to use when we're with babies. According to them, Kari awoke that morning all smiles and the doctor was satisfied that she had recovered from her mysterious illness.

One of the women in the impromptu welcoming committee was a girl I'd graduated from high school with. She told me Kari had the staff wrapped around her little finger. I knew my friend wanted children and I told her maybe she would have a baby of her own some day. She did end up having a little girl, but all was not well with the child. I'll write more on that later.

I had every intention of keeping my promise to God to be more faithful in my church attendance. I made it six Sundays in a row before I began to miss again. Joe is a Catholic and I'm an Episcopalian. We were married in his church and our daughters were baptized there, but I chose not to convert. Sometimes I did feel lonely going to church on my own. Maybe that and having two little ones to take care of in the mornings was part of the reason why I didn't make it every Sunday. But even those excuses didn't stop me from feeling I was letting God down.

My mother came from a long line of Episcopalians. Her parents were both born and raised in England. Her father played the organ and sang in church. There were a couple of priests on my grandmother's side of the family. God is indelibly ingrained in my ancestry and my mother made sure my three brothers and I had every opportunity to know Him in our lives.

We were born in Waukegan, Illinois, but Mom had us christened in her childhood church in Lake Forest. Although we moved to San Francisco, California when I was only five, I do have some vague memories of attending Sunday school and marching around the room singing Onward Christian Soldiers.

Each individual chooses their own level of believing. I think if you have a conscience, you have God. Religion is just a word. Faith is what comes from inside a person. The Bible says faith is being sure of what we hope for and certain of what we do not see.

But I had broken the oath I'd made to God that rainy night in the car, despite my genuine respect for Him. Every Sunday I missed piled on another layer of guilt. I told myself God wouldn't punish me, but a nagging voice inside my head hinted that I just might somehow have to pay for my failure to keep my promise.

I started having a frightening nightmare about Kari when she was eight weeks old. I saw her as a little child in a coffin. She was dead, but I didn't know how she died. Had she been ill? Was she in some kind of accident? My dream never elaborated on any details. How could I protect Kari when I didn't know what I was supposed to be safeguarding her from? Give me a recipe and I'll bake a cake, but present me with something like this and I had no idea what to do.

I'd wake up with tears on my cheeks and scramble out of bed rushing to her crib needing to touch her living warmth. Only then would my heart stop its frantic pounding. I would stand there for long minutes shivering in the middle of the night anxiously watching her gentle breathing.

I wanted to wander happily through carefree flights of fantasy when I slept, not be tormented by eerily realistic portraits of death. Was this a prediction for a heartache that no parent should have to face? Did dreams sometimes come true? The possibility made me feel alienated from myself to realize that such a dreadful thought was housed within my brain.

I'd never studied the significance of dreams and had no idea how to decode them. My dreams were usually of a transient nature, but this one was tenacious enough to make me question its possible validity. It was like having a simple headache that had grown into a full blown migraine. I didn't like it, but the repetition made it difficult to ignore. All I knew was that for some perplexing reason my mind had tormented me with a very callous picture. Was there something wrong with my brain? Had I inherited a flawed gene?

Refusing to accept my dream as a conceivable possibility was my only shield against the disturbing nightmare. No one in their right mind would want to keep something like that rattling around inside their head. I wasn't a psychic. I didn't possess any clairvoyant powers. I finally rationalized that I was an ordinary person who just happened to be having a very unpleasant hallucination in her sleep. I tried to bury my head in the sand, metaphorically speaking, in an effort to block out the terrible image.

I didn't tell anyone about this at the time. I couldn't make the dream stop, but that didn't mean I had to talk about it. I had the nightmare several more times until it suddenly stopped when Kari was still an infant. I thought that was a good sign. I wanted to look forward to a happy, healthy future for my little one as any parent would who loved their child.

We'd had a couple of setbacks with our girls, but everything was fine now. Life was good. I told myself to focus on that and forget about spooky nightmares.

1962 was a year packed with several important historical events. It was quite a year for President John F. Kennedy and the rest of our country. John Glenn went into space on February 20, 1962. Not only was the space program getting a lot of attention, but the Cuban missile crisis came in October of that year.

My parents were living in Key West, Florida at the time, and Mom said all the young Navy wives she'd met were terrified. Who could blame them for being afraid when they were facing the possibility they may be blown up at any time?

Joe and I, with the girls, had driven to Key West in June 1962 to take Mom to her new home. Dad worked for the Navy and had to be there in March. I have to say I was glad we weren't in Florida when Castro decided to point his missiles toward the US.

We had some more family medical concerns in 1962, but not with the girls this time. I had to have a lump removed from my right breast. Thankfully, it was benign. Then Joe's father became ill, and he wasn't so lucky. His diagnoses turned out to be lung cancer.

He'd been a long time heavy smoker like so many men of his generation. No one knew then about the dangers of nicotine. I felt sorry for him. He did so want to become a grandfather, and he loved our girls very much. But now, he might not live to see them grow up. I still recall how he liked to bring them boxes of Cracker Jacks and watch them eagerly digging around the candied popcorn, as they tried to find the little prize inside.

My dad's father died that year in Illinois. I'd only seen my grandfather a couple of times in my life, but there is still that sense of loss. It's a sobering thought to realize that as each generation passes away the next one takes their place. At least that's how I think nature intended it to be; perhaps it should be carved in stone that parents shouldn't be forced to outlive their children.

As 1962 came to a close, life was looking up for our family. The first half of 1963 went well for us. Joe stayed busy with teaching and coaching basketball and baseball at his school. He also belonged to the local Lions Club and got involved with various service projects. I had my own agenda taking care of the girls, attending the Faculty Wives Club, and doing all the necessary daily upkeep in running our household. We even talked about maybe having another child.

Kathy was five-years-old now and so shy that I put her in nursery school for a few hours a week hoping it would help her get ready for kindergarten that coming fall. Kari was two with her own distinctive personality, but she did try to copy pretty much everything Kathy did. She liked animals, dolls, storybooks, and singing. I taught her to sing, *Twinkle, Twinkle Little Star*. She pronounced it, "Tinkle, Tinkle Ittle Tar". She also learned how to sing, *Rock A Bye Baby* in her own special version. It was the cutest thing watching her sitting in a little rocking chair holding a doll and singing, "rock a baby, rock a baby."

The kids and I spent quite a bit of time with my parents that July while Joe was busy with summer work back home. I appreciated having the chance to escape some of the high heat in Oroville for the cooler climate in Napa. My parents had moved back there again when Dad took a job at the Mare Island Naval Shipyard in nearby Vallejo.

13

Mom and I canned applesauce and peaches, poked around in thrift shops, worked jigsaw puzzles, and kept the girls amused with various activities. They loved it when I'd walk with them the couple of blocks to the bus stop, so they could meet my dad after he got off work.

It was a happy, carefree time. I liked spending these days with my mother and seeing how much she enjoyed getting to be around her grandchildren since her return from Florida.

Then August came and our lives slowly began to break apart.

Chapter Two

Kari developed a high fever early in August. I spent most of the night giving her cool sponge baths trying to get her temperature to come down. I called our doctor's office in the morning and was given the name of a new doctor in town. I had no other choice but to make an appointment with him, because my doctor was away on vacation.

The day burned hot as I drove Kari to this new medical office. Temperatures in Oroville often get up into the triple digits during the summer months. I stared through the windshield at the multi-layered strata lining the horizon. A quivering belt of heat hovered just above the asphalt trapping the dust within its shimmering shelf. The pale cloudless sky formed an uninspiring cap for the landscape. Too bad it couldn't rain and clear the air, but that was a remote possibility for this time of year.

I had to wait twenty minutes before I was allowed to take Kari into an examining room, despite the fact that there weren't any other patients in the waiting area. That's a long time when you're holding a sick child who happens to be burning with fever. I could hear the doctor laughing in the background and felt like grinding my teeth at the sound of his gaiety.

The doctor examined Kari and said she had a new virus that was going around. There wasn't any medication for it. The only thing I could do was take her home and keep her as comfortable as possible until the sickness left her body.

I had expected to get more help from him instead of being told her health was essentially in my hands. It was disappointing that he couldn't do anything, but I realized there isn't always a cure-all pill to fix what ails us. I took Kari home and continued with the sponge baths and trying to get her to take liquids. She did start to feel better a couple of days later. But she looked very washed out. Her pallor reminded me of the time when she'd been ill as a baby.

Kari ran another high fever six days later much to my concern. I swear it sounded as though her hair crackled when I touched it. I could easily see her pulse beating rapidly in her neck. Joe and I took her to our doctor, who was back from vacation by then. He said she had swollen tonsils and her ears looked sore. This time I was given an antibiotic for her. I looked at the little bottle and hoped it held some kind of magic elixir inside, powerful enough to make our little girl feel well again.

It didn't work.

I'd given Kari all of the medication, and not only wasn't she feeling better, but her condition had worsened. I called the doctor. He scolded me and said I hadn't given the antibiotic enough time. He also accused me of overreacting. I felt that was unfair. I didn't raise my voice. I wasn't panicky. I just wanted to know what I was supposed to do with my sick child. He said to wait.

I don't know if I'd call it maternal instinct or some kind of inner sense, but I didn't believe the doctor's advice was the best thing for Kari. A mother knows her own child; and when I saw my usually active little girl lying on the sofa after three days, I knew I had to do something to find out why she wasn't improving. But what?

I didn't like going over my doctor's head, but I felt he had let me down. I called a friend who took her children to a pediatrician in the nearby town of Marysville. She gave me his name and office phone number. I wasn't sure if he'd be willing to see Kari without another doctor's referral. But I was given an appointment for her right away when I explained my situation.

Kari was so weak by this time I had to carry her into his office. I'm happy to say I didn't have to wait very long. The first thing the doctor commented on when he saw her was how pale she looked. He said he definitely would want to order some blood tests. I was willing to do anything at this point and agreed. Although he was soft spoken and very gentle while examining her, my poor little girl felt so miserable she cried the whole time.

The doctor called me himself that evening with the results of the tests. He said Kari was very anemic and showed signs of blood loss. That surprised me because I hadn't noticed any visible sign of bleeding. He went on to explain that other symptoms were serious enough to justify a more comprehensive follow up with a specialist.

The last thing he said to me before he hung up was, "At least we know it's not leukemia."

I shuddered at the very mention of the word. The doctor immediately made arrangements for us to take Kari to UC Moffitt Hospital in San Francisco. He also reported his findings to our local doctor, who was still insisting that she'd gotten hold of a tough virus. I have to say I was surprised by his stubbornness because he'd been so quick to call in someone else that time when Kari had the reaction to the nose drops when she was a baby.

Kari was admitted to UC in early October. Kathy had her surgery in San Francisco, but at a different hospital. Thank goodness we now had medical insurance through Joe's job. We hadn't had that luxury for Kathy and ended up having to pay for her operation out of our pocket.

I grew up in San Francisco and had many fond memories of the area. But, this wasn't a very happy way to be returning to the city with another of my children needing medical help.

It turned out to be a very long day including a lot of forms to fill out. I also spent quite a bit of time relating our family history to the doctors assigned to Kari's case. They took copious notes and asked endless questions. It was tedious, but I realized they had to get every scrap of information they could in an effort to help us.

We were finally taken up to the sixth floor pediatric ward, where I undressed Kari for bed. She cried and clung to me while I did the best I could to comfort her. I'd barely gotten her into bed when I was called away to answer more questions. When I returned, Kari was gone, but I could hear her screaming nearby.

My body went rigid as I stood there listening to her cries of distress. She was sick. She was frightened. And I'm sure she must have felt that I had deserted her. What else could Kari think when we'd brought her to this unfamiliar place and subjected her to the care of strangers? I wanted to find her and tell her they were just trying to make her better.

A doctor finally came out of an examining room and told me they were only cleaning out Kari's ears, so they could get a better look. I stayed with her as long as I could when she finally returned to her room. I hoped she would fall asleep, so she wouldn't have to see me leave.

She refused to allow herself to succumb to her weariness even though she was exhausted. I dreaded going and stayed by her bed while she clung to my hand. A nurse finally suggested that Kari might settle down when I was gone. I gave my little girl one last kiss and promised I would see her tomorrow. It took every bit of my willpower not to rush back when I heard her sobbing for me. I hurried down the long hallway and turned the corner for the elevators.

I felt like crying myself. I stepped into the elevator car wondering how many more times I would have to keep leaving one of my children in a hospital. I kept thinking life should be simpler with an even accounting of checks and balances between the good and the bad. The imaginary record book I'd conjured up in my mind had become lopsided against me. It's impossible to explain all the cause and consequences of what happens to us, but in a way we're all searching for the answers.

Kari spent six days at UC while the doctors did several tests, among them a bone marrow test, which we were to come to know and dread.

Kathy and I stayed at my parents' house in Napa. I took her out of school because she was having such a hard time dealing with the newness of kindergarten and with me being away from home. She cried every time I took her to class even after two weeks. Her teacher said she'd never had a student take so long to adjust. I suspected part of Kathy's distress was caused by the turmoil Kari's ill health had brought into our lives.

I can't begin to express how thankful I was that my parents were living in Napa again, as it gave me a comfortable place to stay while Kari was in the hospital. It also helped to have their support during such a trying time. Joe had to stay in Oroville to teach his classes, and I know he appreciated the fact that I didn't have to go through this on my own. But it wasn't easy for him having to be at home waiting and wondering how things were going to turn out.

Mom drove me into the city every day to visit Kari while a neighbor took care of Kathy. Our route took us through what is called the Panhandle of San Francisco's famous Golden Gate Park. We ended up emerging into the Haight Ashbury District. This was the height of the hippie generation of the 1960's. The area had been taken over by people trumpeting their rejection of society's more conventional values. Everywhere we looked there were signs of their particular lifestyle.

It wasn't unusual to see bright blue or shocking purple doors with big yellow sunflowers or fiery red poppies splashed across them. Not surprising when you understood that these were the homes of the flower children, as the residents were dubbed by the media. A few buildings were painted with an outlandish combination of colors. Windows were draped with kaleidoscopic material and macramé, transforming ordinary glass panes into a kind of unique artwork. I must say that driving through the area did help to somewhat brighten up the misery of our trip to the more austere hospital and clinic.

The hospital was located on Paranasus Avenue. I thought the name sounded like some exotic disease. We'd drive up a steep hill, and there at the top was this huge, modern multi-story edifice dominating a large area. A much older building with the dark elaborate architectural style of another era stood adjacent to the hospital.

This was the clinic where patients were sent for their initial visit with doctors and later for outpatient care. The two dissimilar structures standing so close together presented a strange incongruous picture, but each in its own way served a very important purpose. I didn't realize then the vital role those two buildings would play in my future.

Kari was still pretty ill the first three days, but started to feel better on the fourth day and didn't cry when I had to leave her. I was relieved that she'd finally adjusted to her surroundings, but that didn't stop me from carrying a big chunk of guilt away with me every time I had to go. I wanted her home, but mostly I wanted her to be well.

The hospital's pediatric ward had a large colorfully decorated playroom with lots of fun things for the children to do when they felt well enough. Kari loved going there. She was especially fond of painting. She didn't paint pictures; she painted colors. Bright colors went on one page and more subdued colors went on another, until the entire page was completely covered with multi-colored hues. She often painted in the same manner when she was home. I framed some of her artwork and hung them on a wall and kept the rest in a scrapbook.

The doctors released Kari from the hospital, but we were still in limbo as to what was wrong. Her tests weren't conclusive enough for them to give us a definitive diagnosis. They prescribed liquid iron and told us to bring her to the clinic in two weeks for a follow up.

We were happy to have Kari home in time to celebrate her third birthday. My grandmother baked a cake and we had chocolate ice cream, which Kari referred to as her "fabebrit." I did invite some family, but I deliberately wanted to keep the party quiet so there wouldn't be too much excitement for Kari. I bought her a new red dress in hopes it would add some color to her pale cheeks.

The day turned out to be a special occasion for my oldest brother, Boris and wife, Marthine when they announced they were expecting their second child. They already had a daughter who was four months older than Kari. The thought crossed my mind how Joe and I had almost tried for another child. I realized it was probably a good thing we hadn't with Kari's uncertain health.

The little house we were buying at the time was much nicer than the basement apartment we lived in when Kathy was a baby. But I did know it had an eerie bit of history concerning the other two families who'd lived there before us.

The original owners had a three year old girl who died after being hit by a taxi. The next family to move in lost a daughter to spinal meningitis, also at the age of three. I admit I didn't like to think about what happened to those two little girls because here we were with our own three year daughter suffering from an unknown illness.

The house sat on a prime corner lot and was torn down several years after we sold it to an elderly woman. A Walgreens store is there now. The older daughter of the original owners told me she thought the house was cursed.

Kari seemed to be improving. I could hear her laughter, as she ran around playing with Kathy. Her appetite was better and she'd gained back some of the weight she'd lost. I thought the crisis had passed and felt some of my anxiousness begin to disappear.

It turned out to be a short-lived reprieve. Her fever came back a week later, and the little energy she gained quickly dwindled away.

The girls and I went back to Napa. Mom and my second oldest brother, Grant drove us for Kari's first visit to the UC outpatient clinic. I was glad to have their company. It turned out to be another long, frustrating day. I filled out endless forms again, stood in lines, and waited and waited. Most of the personnel treated me politely enough. But the woman I had to meet with concerning our financial status and medical insurance was downright unpleasant.

I realized it was her job to make sure the clinic received payment, but surely she could have shown a little more respect for my situation. I certainly didn't relish being there. I wore a simple knit dress from a Penney's sale catalog. The woman said she hoped my insurance would kick in, so I wouldn't have to end up dressing in rags. Like Shakespeare's Shylock, she wanted her pound of flesh. I wished I had the quick wit to fire back with a quick salvo, but I've never been good at that kind of thing.

At least the doctor I had to meet with turned out to be nice. He was young and quiet spoken.

Our paths would cross many times over the next three years. I later read how important his contributions were in the medical world, particularly with bone marrow transplants.

Kari had to go through another round of blood work and examinations. She spent most of the day in tears from being poked and prodded so much. Finally, I was called into a large room at the end of the day. Several doctors were sitting in a semicircle. I can still recall two of them very well because I saw them several times after that initial meeting. They were pediatric hematologists in charge of the clinic.

Their age and distinguished manner reminded me of the doctor who had performed Kathy's surgery. They exuded that same kind of professionalism and genuine empathy that made me feel as though Kari's wellbeing was as special to them as it was to me.

They told me the liquid iron I'd been giving her hadn't helped to improve the anemia. I wasn't surprised. I only had to look at her prolonged paleness to know that myself. They wanted me to bring her back to the clinic in a week for another bone marrow and blood work. I felt myself inwardly wince at the thought of Kari having to go through all that again. Reluctantly, the girls and I stayed at my parents' home, and Joe came to see us on the weekend.

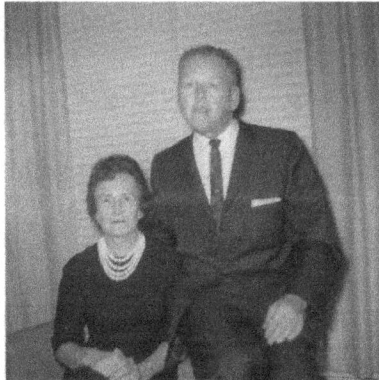

Grandma & Grandpa Brown

Kari began to complain of headaches and a stiff neck, in addition to running a fever. I loved my sweet child. She was everything a mother could ask for. Now I began to worry that perhaps the doctors might not be able to make her well. I hated myself for such a repugnant thought, but sometimes our minds take us where we don't want to go.

October 29, 1963; ordinarily I'd be at home getting ready for Halloween. I should have been setting out decorations, buying trick or treat candy, and putting the final touches on the girls' costumes. Instead, I sat in a car heading back to the clinic in San Francisco with my mother and Kari. The hippie peace signs I spotted everywhere as we drove through their domain conflicted with the sense of uneasiness I was feeling.

At the clinic, the same young doctor we'd met before examined Kari. He asked me how she'd felt during the last week. I described what had been going on and watched his reaction for signs of alarm; but his expression remained passive. He made arrangements for her bone marrow and blood work.

After the tests were completed, the staff told us to take Kari upstairs to the fifth floor and wait outside one of the rooms there. Mom and I sat on a long wooden bench, worn smooth probably by countless other people. The afternoon was slowly wearing away. I looked up and down the long corridor and saw that we were the only ones in the area. It was eerily quiet compared to the hustle and bustle we'd been surrounded with all morning downstairs.

Why weren't there any other people here? Were we being isolated? If so, why? I'd already been fighting my nervousness, but now my stomach began to squeeze into a hard knot. Mom and I didn't talk too much because we didn't want to disturb Kari as she dozed on my mother's lap.

The same doctor finally came down the hallway and summoned me into a small room. He closed the door and asked me to sit down before he pulled another chair around to face me. There wasn't much light coming in through the one narrow window, so he flicked on a light switch.

My heart began to jump around like a stone bouncing off a hard surface when I saw his hands shake. He opened the folder he'd been carrying. I'd seen it before and knew it held the results of Kari's medical tests.

At first, he just stared down at the paperwork in front of him. He finally looked at me, and I held my breath at his expression. He actually looked grief stricken. He told me Kari's anemia was worse, but she had something far more serious.

Here it comes, I thought, and braced myself. When he said the words, acute leukemia, I stared at him and waited for a glimmer of hope that I might have misunderstood him. But he looked as solemn as I felt.

Then, in a sudden blinding flashback, I remembered my nightmare. Was this a dreadful coincidence, or had that dream actually been prophetic?

"Are you saying that my Kari has no more tomorrows?" I finally managed to utter.

I guess that sounded pretty melodramatic, but those are the words that popped out of my mouth.

He nodded.

"We suspected what she had right from the beginning, but we hoped we would be proven wrong. Today's bone marrow confirmed the diagnosis."

He explained that Kari had to be hospitalized immediately where she would be started on a course of treatment. There were five drugs available to treat the disease. They could help her live from possibly nine months to a year. Part of my brain was trying to understand what he was saying, but another part was rebelling against this death knell he was delivering.

I can't even begin to describe how sick I felt inside. My heart was pounding so hard by this time that it actually hurt my chest. I just sat there staring at him unable for the moment to form another coherent sentence. The doctor shifted on his chair and cleared his throat.

"Would you like me to tell your mother?" he asked in his quiet voice.

Although it wasn't something I was looking forward to, I felt I should be the one to break such devastating news to my mom. I shook my head and somehow found the will to talk.

"No, that's all right. I'll do it."

The doctor went on to tell me that he would go and make the necessary arrangements to admit Kari to the hospital. Then he would send a nurse for us when everything was ready. A panicky voice inside my head kept yelling this had to be a mistake.

He stood up and reached for the door handle, pausing for a moment to look at me again.

"I'm so very sorry, Mrs. High."

I nodded, too miserable to speak. Rules and regulations fetter us all, some more difficult than others to obey, but we sometimes have the freewill to accept or reject them. That option wasn't available to me now. Kari had a life threatening disease, and I couldn't change that.

I followed him out the door and watched him quickly disappear down the corridor before I turned toward my mother. I felt myself falter and had to force my shaky legs to move. Kari was still asleep. She reminded me of a delicate little princess in her pretty blue and white dress and white patent leather shoes with the lace trimmed socks.

"I saw the doctor leave," Mom said. "What did he say? Is it all right to take Kari home?"

She had to ask me three times before I was able to answer her. I struggled for composure, because I knew if I started to cry I might not be able to stop.

Chapter Three

"Don't you know? Can't you guess?" I said in a quivering voice I barely recognized as my own. "It's the very worst thing we were afraid might be wrong. Kari has leukemia."

I heard my mother's swift intake of breath and saw the look of disbelief flit across her face.

"Oh, no!" she cried before she got up and walked over to a row of windows.

She held Kari in her arms. Mom was only a little over five feet tall and Kari was kind of big for her to be carrying, but I didn't go to them. I stood riveted to my own patch of floor, engulfed in an overwhelming sense of sorrow. The reality was more horrible than my nightmare.

A nurse came to take us over to the hospital. I carefully lifted Kari from my mother's arms. She barely stirred, as I held her against me. We trailed behind the nurse, as she navigated the twists and turns of several corridors leading to the pediatric ward.

Kari woke up as I undressed her and put her in a hospital gown. It was yellow with little animals printed on it. Another nurse brought in a dinner tray. I sat with Kari at a little table in her room trying to help her eat. But she was still too drowsy from the sedative she'd been given before the bone marrow test to take more than a few bites of the food.

I picked her up and carried her over to the bed. I'd just finished tucking her in when one of the doctors from her previous stay motioned me to join her in the hallway. She told me she was very sorry and prayed it wouldn't come to this. We stood there talking for a few minutes while medical personnel passed by going about their duties.

Life ebbed and flowed all around me while I felt like my world was collapsing. Kari was sleeping deeply when I returned to her room. I gently brushed aside a few strands of hair that had fallen across her face and bent down to kiss her on one pallid cheek. I stood there looking at my precious little girl through a blur of sadness. I barely noticed a nurse coming into the room until she spoke.

"We'll take good care of her for you, Mrs. High," she said in a soft voice.

I thanked her and took one last look at Kari before I turned and left the room. I kept thinking this kind of thing happened to other people, not to me. But it really was happening to me. My heart was swollen with anguish and my body felt curiously heavy like I was carrying heavy weights.

Mom and I left the hospital and headed for her car. You don't measure a walk like that in time or distance, but rather in heartbeats. I wondered how many steps I'd be able to take because my legs felt like they wanted to crumble beneath me.

My mother had called my dad to tell him the news before we left the hospital. I don't even remember the drive back to Napa. Dad met us at the door of their house, but didn't say much. I was glad because I wasn't ready to talk about things right then.

I forced myself to eat some of the dinner he'd prepared. My father was a good cook, but I could have been eating straw for all I knew. I sat with my parents and stared at the television program even though I didn't have a clue what I was watching.

Joe telephoned as we'd planned. I told him to brace himself for some really awful news. He was stunned and asked if there was a cure. When I told him no, he wanted to know how long Kari would be able to last with such a serious illness. I repeated what the doctor had told me. We were too upset to say more and bid each other a very sad goodnight.

I worried about Joe being home alone, but he told me later that my aunt and uncle invited him to their house for a while when he called to tell them about Kari's diagnosis. He also called his parents and a few of our close friends before he just couldn't bear to talk about it anymore. He told me he cried after he went to bed.

He wasn't the only one to shed tears that night.

I crawled into bed while my parents stood in the doorway of the bedroom. We'd avoided talking about what was happening, but my dad finally broke the silence.

"I'm so sorry. You know your mother and I would give anything not to have this happen to our little Kari."

It's easy to be conquered by weakness in such a heartbreaking situation. His words triggered the tears I'd been fighting for the last few hours. He came into the room to try and comfort me, but ended up crying himself. My mother stood in the doorway, sobbing. In between my own sobs I kept saying how much I loved Kari and that I didn't want to be left with just a gravestone.

Again, I know that sounds pretty dramatic, but I doubt if anyone knows what they'll say under such dire circumstances. All I could think about was that my beautiful little girl was going to die. My head throbbed from crying, and it felt as though a steel band squeezed my chest.

Kathy was in the same room and slept through everything. I felt glad of that because I'm sure seeing all the adults crying would have been very upsetting for her. My dad offered me a sleeping pill. I'm not a pill popper, but I knew I probably wasn't going to get much sleep without taking something. It did help and I managed to get some rest.

Did I think God was punishing me? Of course I did. I'm as superstitious as the next person. I felt that he had betrayed me despite the fact I was the one who hadn't kept my vow. I eventually came to realize that it was not so much a sense of faithlessness or lack of trust that made me think I was being penalized by God, but simply a characteristic of being human.

I could have continued to blame Him, but what good would that do me?

Kathy asked me why Kari wasn't there when I awoke the next morning. I told her she was sick and had to stay in the hospital, but would be coming home as soon as she felt better.

"Can I go see her?" she wanted to know.

"No, honey, I'm sorry, but the hospital rules won't let you."

Her bottom lip immediately started to wobble and the beginning of tears welled up. I put my arms around her.

"Why don't you draw Kari a nice picture and I'll take it to her?"

She sniffed and nodded.

"Okay."

Joe was too depressed to teach the next day. He came to Napa to take Kathy and me home with him. It felt good to be home even for a little while. Kathy knew Halloween was coming and I didn't want to deny her the chance to enjoy herself. Her life had already been thrown out of sync enough these last couple of months. Friends invited us to dinner and I took Kathy trick or treating with their two sons. I was in a bowling league at the time and it was my team's night to bowl. I'd never been very athletic, but ironically enough I had my highest series that night since I began to bowl. I hardly remembered it. I was moving around like a zombie in a fog. I'd get up, throw the ball down the alley, and then sit down until it was my turn again. I felt as wilted as a leaf of week-old lettuce. My thoughts were so engrossed thinking about Kari's diagnosis that my sudden expertise meant absolutely nothing to me.

We returned to the hospital the next day. I felt such a relief to see Kari looking and feeling so much better. I began to hope that the doctors were mistaken about her having leukemia. Joe and I visited with her for awhile before one of the head pediatric hematologists I'd met in the big conference room at the clinic asked to speak to us in private. We followed him into a small room. He introduced himself to Joe and invited us to sit down.

He explained that it'd been so difficult diagnosing Kari because she was in such early stages of the disease. The kind of leukemia she had was rare, affecting something like one in 100,000 people. Her blood stream was full of leukemic cells, as her platelets, white blood cells, and red blood cells were affected.

The doctor said it would be like walking into a football stadium and having one side all wearing red and people on the other side all being dressed in blue. He couldn't have put it anymore succinctly than that. There could be no mistaking what Kari had. So much for my fantasy that a mistake had been made.

Joe and I sat there listening as the doctor took us through the depressing facts. Kari may appear well at times, but he emphasized there was no cure and cautioned us not to be fooled by claims to the contrary. We found out later why he was so careful to point that out when people started sending us articles on so-called miracle cures. One claimed a daily glass of tomato juice would cure leukemia. I wasn't an expert, but that sounded utterly preposterous.

The doctor went on to explain that Kari might stay feeling well for a few weeks, or if she responded to the drugs and went into remission, she could go on for months. Any longevity beyond that would be the exception, not the rule. He said he thought she could live, with luck, twelve to fifteen months. I couldn't help thinking at least he'd predicted a few more months than I'd been told earlier.

Kathy's lip had been taken care of pretty easily. But there wasn't going to be any way to fix Kari's problem. The grim prospect meant we could lose her soon after she turned four.

We came to learn that remissions were little dashes of pseudo cures that tantalize you with periods of false hope. They became the islands of haven in the turbulent sea of the disease. They're the flat stones to jump on as you pass over a raging stream, but when you look back, they've disappeared. We ended up having to jump a little further each time, and the stones became smaller, leaving us floundering.

Joe and I went back to Kari's room after the doctor finished talking to us. We had to do some pretty great acting, as we smiled and tried to stay cheerful for our little girl when we were hurting so bad inside we ached. Once again, leaving her was very hard. She cried, begging us to take her home. I hated those departures. They cut into me, whittling away at my spirit, making me feel raw and miserable. I wanted to weep for my family and myself, but mostly for Kari.

Joe and Kathy had to go home the next day to return to school. She began to cry when she realized I wouldn't be going with them. I hugged her and promised to come home just as soon as I could. It was an emotional tug of war for me. I wanted to be with both my little girls, but I had to make a choice and stay with Kari. I stood in front of my parent's house and watched Joe drive away with Kathy's tearful face staring at me from the window.

Kari was released from the hospital on November 4th. She and I took the bus to Oroville after spending the night at my parents' house. The last of the warm weather had drifted away, chilling the air and leaving the sky gray with heavy mists. But it may as well been a bright sunny day as far as she was concerned. She was in a jovial mood, happy to be going home.

Riding the Greyhound Bus was a new and exciting adventure for Kari. She watched the passing scenery commenting every time she saw something that interested her. I let her wear the plastic bracelets I had on. She dropped one and it rolled under the seat in front of us, out of reach. I told her it was all right. I still have the rest of that set of bracelets to this day.

Joe and Kathy met us at the bus station. Kari ran to him and shrieked with delight when he swept her up into his arms. Kathy's greeting was more subdued than I expected. I had the feeling that she was trying to decide if her little sister really was well enough before she touched her. Kari wasn't worried. She ran over and gave her big sister a heartfelt hug.

The friends who'd invited us to their house and had Kathy go trick or treating with their two sons asked us to dinner that night. Kari thought this was a wonderful way to welcome her home and couldn't wait to join the boys in their games. Looking at them, she appeared just as healthy as they did. What a sweet delusion.

It's not easy for a parent to have their child be seriously ill. My parents certainly understood this. I was born with a digestive problem and came very close to dying in infancy. I weighed one ounce over five pounds at birth and soon began to lose weight because I couldn't take in nourishment. I had to be fed barley water through an eyedropper every fifteen minutes. My mother had to dress me in doll clothes and carry me around on a pillow because I was so fragile.

I knew from the things they told me that my illness caused them great distress. Mom said they took me to several doctors who said nothing could be done. My father pleaded with the last doctor not to send me home to die. That man was the one who came up with the idea to try the barley water. I'm alive today thanks to that last ditch effort and my parent's devotion.

Now I was the parent filled with a sense of helplessness. All I could think about was losing Kari. I forgot all the things that were good in my life because I kept centering on this one terrible event. My friend's advice about being happy that Kathy's lip could be fixed didn't apply here. This wasn't something plastic surgery could repair. I knew I had to give up the idea that my family should have been spared this calamity, but I did feel like life was being unfair.

Kari was so full of pep and looked so healthy, how could she have leukemia? Her color was good and she was running around. I tried to fan a little flicker of optimism, despite what the doctors told us. Mistakes were made in the medical field. My mind grappled with what I'd been told and with what I saw when I looked at Kari. No wonder we were warned not to be deceived. But the heart knows what it wants to believe.

You can be as rich as Croesus, but no matter how much money you have, it can't buy you complete immunity from every catastrophe. My Aunt June called me on November 22, 1963, crying. I worried something awful must had happened to her or someone in her family. I had a difficult time understanding her because she was so upset, but she finally managed to ask me if I had my TV on. I told her no and she urged me to turn it on right away before she hung up.

I didn't get the chance to ask her what channel I was supposed to use, but as soon as I turned on the set, it didn't matter. The terrible news event was being broadcast on every station with the grisly details of President Kennedy's assassination. I sat watching in disbelief over the next several days along with millions of others. I don't think I'll ever forget the sight of little John-John Kennedy's salute to his fallen father, as the funeral cortege slowly rolled by with the president's coffin.

This was what I meant earlier about these two little children being born in the same year and both having tragedy strike their lives in 1963.

Kari had to be taken to the clinic for weekly visits. I became acquainted with some of the other parents whose children were also receiving treatment. It was heartbreaking to see how many there were. Most of them were around Kari's age, but one of the boys was an older thirteen-year-old. He'd been diagnosed a couple of months before Kari.

He was a good looking young man with dark wavy hair and a sprinkling of freckles across his nose. His name was Larry. Somehow, he and Kari were drawn toward each other, despite their age difference. He had unending patience with her and she adored him. Mom and I befriended his mother. She was older than all us other parents.

Although we were an eclectic group from varying backgrounds, we developed a kind of kinship amongst ourselves. The clinic was a world away from where we wanted to be. We were thrown together by the common denominator of our children sharing the same illness.

Humans are normally social and tend to instinctively gravitate towards one another seeking comfort in times of crisis. We should have worn badges stating the date of our child's diagnosis because that was usually the first question we'd ask each other. I suppose we were trying to get an idea how long our child would live by comparing the dates with the other kids.

We found ourselves speaking this strange new vocabulary connected with the disease. Words like remission, bone marrow, hematology, platelets, red blood cells, white blood cells, anemia, hemorrhage, and other terms not normally used in every-day language. The disease victimizes the parents as much as the children; just in a different way.

Family and friends can empathize with you, but they can't understand what you're truly feeling. Those of us sitting in the clinic or the hospital with our sick children had become somewhat segregated from more fortunate parents who weren't being forced to go through our ordeal.

The first drug the doctors put Kari on gave her a ravenous appetite. She wanted to eat all the time. I'd put her to bed at night and she'd get up asking for more food. She gained a lot of weight rapidly and became very bloated, especially in her face and stomach. I had to buy her larger size clothes.

It was December, and I told her she looked like Santa Claus. The doctors were pleased that I was trying to use humor to elevate the situation, but they also apologized for the way the drug had distorted Kari's usually dainty body. I would come to learn that each drug came with its own side effects, as the potential benefits competed with a wide range of risks. The drugs gave her a measure of relief from the leukemia, but not without making her put up with something unpleasant in return.

Kari enjoyed preparing for Christmas. Joe bought the girls a little tree for their bedroom and I put a string of colored lights on it. She'd sit at her little red table singing Christmas carols while cutting out old Christmas cards making decorations. Kathy would help when she wasn't in school. Kari also got her hands into the cookie dough and colored sugar while helping me decorate cutout cookies. She helped wrap presents and put up ornaments around the house. She wanted to be a part of everything.

One very special part of my Christmas since I was a child is an old cardboard manger. It was a gift from neighbors to my family in 1944, and our last Christmas in Illinois. I may not put up as many decorations now as I used to, but that manger always comes out of its box.

Our family and friends showered Kathy and Kari with gifts that year. I think in their own way they were trying to show us how much they wanted to do something for the girls. The children were especially elated with the talking dolls from friends and the lovely white fur hats and matching muffs from Joe's mother.

Kari was so happy. She laughed a lot and told us several times a day how much she loved us. She enjoyed "playing the piano" and making up songs to go with her picture books. The girls also had a small record player in their bedroom and Kari was particularly fond of playing the record, *London Bridges* that month. We read to her quite a bit and her favorite story at that time was *The Sword in the Stone*. She began memorizing nursery rhymes when she was two and could recite quite a few by herself. Music and stories were an important part of her life.

Joe bought a swing set with a slide and glider in February 1964. Kari insisted she needed to "*help*" daddy put it together. She couldn't wait to hop on as soon as it was finished. She quickly learned how to pump herself on the swings.

"Look at me, I'm big now," she proudly announced.

She loved to sit on the glider with Kathy. If her sister wasn't there, Kari would take her dolls or a stuffed animal and sit them in the glider with her. She'd swing back and forth, singing all the songs she could remember and others she made up. She liked the slide, too, and usually went down on her tummy.

The doctors let her go two weeks in between clinic visits after she had several good lab reports. I appreciated not having to go so often, especially because it was so heart wrenching to see the other sick children. There was often someone going through a bad time. One of the little boys was screaming on one of our visits because he was in so much pain before the medical staff could help him. I couldn't help but pity his anguished parents.

We never knew when Kari would end up with a bad report. Her liver was enlarged in March and her red blood cell count was down, so she had to have another bone marrow test. It turned out to be an awful day in more ways than one. Kathy came home from school with the chicken pox. So besides having to have sedation shots for the bone marrow and two blood tests, Kari also had to have chicken pox gamma globulin.

Mom was with me that clinic day. She had to walk away because she couldn't bear to listen to Kari's screams. I held Kari trying to comfort her. I felt like I was fracturing into a million tiny pieces. I don't think there's anything worse than having to watch a little child suffering and not be able to do anything about it. She was so exhausted from this latest trauma that she slept for ten hours straight.

The month of March ended up being a very trying month. The chicken pox didn't hit Kathy very hard, but she did have a persistent infection in her mouth. Joe and Kari both ended up getting the chicken pox. It happened during his week spring break from school, but he had to take off an extra week because he was so sick. They were both absolutely miserable.

He literally paced the floor, and she cried because she itched so badly. I called her doctors at UC and they prescribed medication to help relieve her itching and something else to help her sleep. I had to call our doctor for Joe, and he actually came to our house. He took one look at Joe and said it was the worst case of chicken pox he'd ever encountered.

I wasn't getting much rest taking care of everyone else and ended up getting a sore throat, headache, and nausea for five days. My mother came to take care of us.

Easter came in March that year, but no one felt up to going to church or celebrating in any way.

Kari did get a good report at her next clinic visit, despite all the illness we'd had in the family. The doctors put her on a different medication for the leukemia and she went back to her normal weight. The poor little thing hated those painful finger pricks necessary for her routine blood work. The ladies in the lab were always so sweet, and I never failed to see the sympathy in their eyes when they'd gently hold Kari's hand in theirs.

"We'll be real fast, Kari," they'd tell her.

We took Kari to Kathy's kindergarten play, *The Little Red Hen*, in June of 1964, just before school was out for the summer. She enjoyed it so much she begged me to let her go back to Kathy's classroom. I told her she had to be five years old to go to kindergarten. She held up her hand and wiggled her five fingers.

"When will I be this many, Mommy?"

I told Kathy's teacher how much Kari liked being at school. She was nice enough to let Kari spend the next afternoon in class. That same woman was buying a house in southern California a few years later and Kathy's godfather happened to be the appraiser. He mentioned us when he found out she'd taught in Oroville. He told us later that she remembered Kathy and the ill little sister who was so eager to go to school.

Kari had a good clinic report in June and felt quite perky on the drive home. She sang, *Don't Sit Under the Apple Tree,* and *Take Me Out to the Ballgame.* She especially liked to put heavy emphasis on the word, *root.* It started to rain as we pulled into our driveway. She pointed to the drops of water.

"Look! The ground has the chicken pops."

She was such a little character. Joe brought the girls a wading pool. Kari was playing in it one hot afternoon and saw that a bird had left a deposit on one of the floating toys. I had a feeling she would make a comment when I saw her pick it up.

"Hey, somebody went bird potty on Kathy's toy."

Sadness mingled with the good times. One of the boys we'd met at the clinic passed away that month. Death was always lurking in the shadows ready to grab these children. The best we parents could do was to take each day as they came and hope for a better tomorrow. It wasn't easy. We'd see one of the children at the clinic and then suddenly rumors would circulate that they were gone. The reality of these deaths was particularly harsh because it involved little kids.

August became a nightmare for us that stretched into September. Kari was anemic, and her liver was enlarged again. The doctors had to put her on another drug because she was having a relapse. She developed a fever and began to complain of stomach aches. I took her to the pediatrician in Marysville. He prescribed medication, but her pain persisted for the next two days. She ended up having to go back to UC.

It was a hot summer day. I stared out the car window, as Joe drove us out of town. Days of relentless scorching sun had sucked all the moisture out of the land. The ground reminded me of old tan suede, worn and lackluster. Dust and billowing smoke from nearby grass fires mingled, rising up to foul the air. San Francisco's cooler climate was a blessed relief.

I wish I could have said the same thing about Kari's condition. She was diagnosed with *peritonitis poisoning*.

The doctors put her on antibiotics fed intravenously through a vein in her arm, but she was so restless she pulled the needle out. The same thing happened when they tried the other arm. They tried oral medication after that.

Kari sobbed when we had to leave. Joe said it made him feel physically ill when he walked away with the sound of her cries echoing down the hallway after us. I certainly knew what he was going through.

The oral medicine didn't help her, and she was put back on the IV. Kari's hands were tied down in hopes of keeping the needle in place. I knew this was to help her, but sometimes medical treatments seem almost as awful as the illness.

She was screaming the next day when I hurried into her room.

"Mommy! Mommy! I want my Mommy!"

She sounded terribly hoarse, as though she'd been crying for quite a while. Pain and drugs had robbed her eyes of their sparkle. An incision had been made in her leg now, so a tube could be inserted up into a vein for the antibiotics. Patches of her skin were scaled from tape and her arms were red and puffy. Veins in her hands, arms, and feet bore pockmarks from needles.

My heart ached, as I stood there looking at her. I can't stand the thought of any child suffering for whatever reason. Having to experience this with my own daughter made it even worse.

Were we doing the right thing to put her through all this? I wanted to relieve Kari of her suffering, but now I felt as though we were making things worse.

Chapter Four

Kari did begin to show improvement after this procedure. She also had to have a couple of blood transfusions before we were finally allowed to bring her home. It had been a harrowing sixteen days and her misery wasn't over yet. Somehow no one noticed that the stitches to close the incision in her leg hadn't been removed when they took the tube out. I took the bandage off a couple of days later and could see that the incision was beginning to fester. Joe and I had to take her to our hospital's emergency room.

The drug Kari was on now was too toxic to take in pill form. She had to get the drug by injection. Her UC doctors made arrangements for the pediatrician in Marysville to do this, so we wouldn't have to drive to San Francisco every time. I didn't realize Kari had come into the kitchen while I was calling to make the appointment until I heard her start to cry.

She understood what injection meant by now. She pleaded with me not to make her have any more shots. Then she begged me not to leave her at the doctor's office. I knelt down and put my arms around her. It must have seemed to this poor child that the person she should most be able to trust had systematically gone about repeatedly subjecting her to pain. I was beginning to feel like an ogress.

The doctors advised us not to tell Kari she wasn't going to get well because it would be too frightening for her. It wasn't easy coming up with reasons why she had to suffer so much, but who would want to tell a four-year-old child that they were going to die?

Kari started to feel better the end of September and she received an encouraging report at her clinic visit. The doctors felt that she was strong enough to be taken off the injections and tolerate her drug in pill form. She never complained having to take so many pills. I'd say it wasn't too surprising now that she knew about the more unpleasant ways to get her medicine.

Joe had his birthday in mid-September and I baked him a cake. Once again we tried to weave ourselves back into the fabric of our daily lives. A normal routine can be comforting and you don't realize how much you miss it until everything familiar has been taken away.

We gave Kari a small party in mid October for her fourth birthday. I was glad she enjoyed this little celebration and that we still had her with us. But her unstable health never allowed us to relax for very long. That's the sword that hangs over your head when you're dealing with an incurable illness. Anything, no matter how minor it may seem, could be something significant and had to be thoroughly examined.

I knew it wasn't unusual for children to experience any number of maladies in childhood. It's all part of growing up. Unfortunately, in Kari's case we were forced to be overly vigilant because of the leukemia. Maybe I was beginning to sound like a hypochondriac on my daughter's behalf, but she was very vulnerable to just about any germ that came her way. What choice did I have when a simple cough could turn into something as serious as pneumonia?

A few days after her birthday Kari vomited, had headaches, and complained of a stiff neck. The doctors had forewarned me that this could mean the disease was going to her brain. We ended up taking her to the clinic where she had to have a spinal tap. It turned out to be clear, but I couldn't keep myself from cringing at the sound of her screaming. It's the kind of feeling you get when you hear someone dragging their fingers over a chalkboard. I had the strongest urge to put my hands over my ears.

Kari ended October and started November with more vomiting. Her doctors thought at one point that she might have the flu. She did get to go trick or treating that year. She wore a bunny costume. I realized she'd gotten through the one year mark since her diagnosis, but at such a terrible cost to her frail little body.

I'll never know how she still managed to keep her sense of humor considering all she was going through. She liked to look at a picture of herself taken when she was five months old. Her hair was tousled in the photo.

"Can I see the picture of me with my hair flopped up?" she'd ask.

I love that photo and have it hanging in our house in a collage of family pictures.

One time after she'd finished washing her hands, she brought them out of the towel, waved her fingers in front of her face and said, "Well, hello there."

Kari decided she should stand up going to the bathroom when a friend visited us one day with her little boy and Kari got a peek at him doing his business. I explained to her that only boys went to the bathroom that way.

She looked down at herself.

"Oh. I guess my tinkler got smashed."

Her cute sayings continue to amuse us all. My brother, Grant was out of the Army at this time and working as a plumber's helper. One day he was visiting us and Kari asked why he wasn't plumbing. He told her it was his day off.

"Well, you'd better get busy because those plums need to get picked, Uncle Grant."

One night I was getting Kari ready to go to bed and I knew she wanted to stay up.

"Mommy, do you know how to say 'tired' in German?"

I told her I didn't, so she rattled over some gibberish.

Then she said, "Do you know how to say I'm not sleepy and don't want to go to bed, in German?"

I busted up laughing.

She loved making up silly little jokes. Example: "Who puts bellybuttons in his nose?"

We'd have to guess different animals until we came to one that suited her.

We received the good news in her December clinic visit that Kari was in remission again. That's how it was with remissions. Our lives yo-yoed up and down according to when she was able to sustain the "quiet periods" as the doctors called them. We relished those times with the fervor of a dog enjoying a prize bone because it was all we had.

Other things happened that clinic day. Kari's blood work showed that she was missing a globulin fraction. It has something to do with how a person fights off illness. Joe, Kathy, and I each had a vial of blood drawn that day, but ours came out normal.

We saw Larry the same day. He didn't look well and ended up being put in the hospital. I also heard that a little boy Kari used to play with at the clinic had died just before Thanksgiving.

That shocked me because he looked so healthy just two weeks ago. Life became transitory for these children at a young age because of the leukemia. They were here for a short time and then they left for another world. We could only hope for a gentler, kinder existence for them. They'd certainly earned the privilege to be in a place free from pain and disease.

Despite her good report in early December, Kari spent most of the month suffering from fever, a cough, and an ear infection. She acted very subdued and would barely talk to us. Bedtime became especially difficult. It wasn't like the times when she just wasn't sleepy. Now she acted almost panicky when I'd put her in bed. I had to sit with her until she fell asleep.

She may not have understood what was happening to her, but her body felt the pain and discomfort of her illness. I was somewhat surprised at this abrupt change in her behavior because she acted so excited at Christmas opening her gifts and playing with Kathy. Kari especially enjoyed the aqua blue peddle car we gave her. She had fun riding it on our patio when the weather was good and her legs didn't ache.

She also received a gift that Christmas that would distinguish itself in a very special way.

One of Joe's boyhood friends was a Catholic priest. Joe wrote and asked him to pray for Kari when we learned she had leukemia. The man told his mother about Kari and the woman sent her a beautiful miniature statue of the Virgin Mary. She had a long, flowing white dress and a blue robe with gold trim. A tiny halo crown encrusted with sparkling blue stones encircled her head.

Kari was enthralled with this figurine. She ended up holding it every night at bedtime when she was home and made up this prayer: *"Virgin Mary, make me better, so everyone will think I'm better."*

Kari didn't want people to think of her as being sick. She just wanted to be a normal little girl. Sometimes the music of one's life is lost in the torment of the soul, compromised by what we have no control over. But I don't think she understood the concept of giving up. Her basic instinct was to survive.

Kari did start 1965 with a good blood report, although she had another ear infection and a couple of nasty sores in her mouth. Those sores were caused by the toxic drugs she was taking, so her doctors decided to try a different combination. What a day it turned out to be. Kari vomited down the front of my black dress while Mom drove us to San Francisco. I did my best to clean us both up in the restroom as soon as we arrived at the clinic.

Our trip home was even worse.

My mother's car began to overheat. Steam was billowing out of the radiator by the time we approached the tollbooth at the Bay Bridge. They stopped all traffic and had her drive across the front of the booths to a maintenance building.

A man added water, and we started on our way again. We didn't get very far when the car started to heat up again. Mom took an off ramp hoping to find a service station, but the only one we saw was closed for the night. Luckily, we found a truck terminal nearby, and the men there were very helpful.

I felt thankful that Kari had fallen asleep on the backseat. It was pouring rain and inky black out. The car's tires made a hissing sound on the wet asphalt and the many reflections from the oncoming headlights were almost blinding. My mom sat hunched over the wheel, staring straight ahead, concentrating on her driving. I worried for her having to drive in such awful conditions.

And then my body suddenly began to tighten up like the skin on a drum until my hands and arms went completely numb. My fingers curled into claws and I couldn't straighten them out. I didn't know why this was happening to me and I was scared. But I didn't say anything to my mother. She had enough to worry about just trying to get us home safely. Thank goodness I was all right by the time we arrived at her house.

I thought about my strange reaction later and the only thing I could come up with was that I'd been so nervous it had somehow affected my body in this way. That's not too surprising because I have a tendency to be a nervous sort even when things are going well, and things were definitely not going well that night.

I worried about Kari being on her own so much because she was often too ill to play with other children, and Kathy was in school all day. My parents came up with the idea to buy her a dog. It seemed like the logical thing to do because she really loved animals. We knew it would have to be a very gentle dog with a lot of patience, as Kari's lifestyle was becoming more and more sedentary as her illness progressed.

Mom saw an ad in the Napa newspaper for a white, female, four month-old miniature poodle. We found out the other puppies from the litter were already gone, but this one had been the runt of the group and required some extra care.

The owners named her Cuddles and that pretty much summoned up the kind of dog she turned out to be.

She had such a placid nature we couldn't have asked for a pet more suited to Kari's needs. Child and dog instantly hit it off.

That little animal never strayed very far from Kari's side when she was home. If Kari felt well enough to play, then Cuddles would play with her. When she wasn't having a good day, Cuddles would stay next to her for as long as she was needed.

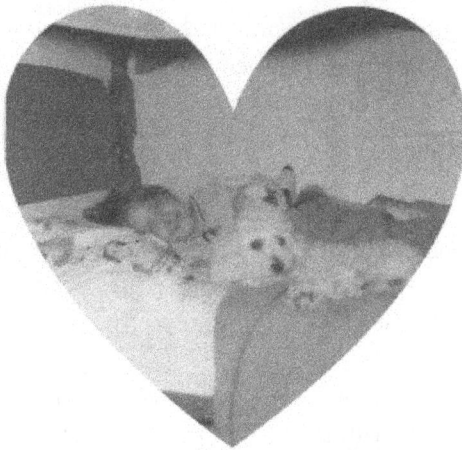

Cuddles keeping Kari company in bed

I'd read stories and watched movies about this kind of devotion between children and their pets, but this was the first time I had ever witnessed such a thing firsthand. A person just had to see the two of them together to know how touching their bond had become.

February turned out to be another hellish month. Kari had headaches and vomited several times. I phoned her pediatrician and he advised me to call UC. I was able to contact one of her hematologists at his private practice and explained what was happening. He said some of the leukemia cells had probably gotten into her spine. He reminded me they would cause brain damage if left unchecked. He told me to take her to the hospital right away.

I immediately called Joe at school and then made arrangements with my aunt to take care of Kathy. I dashed off a quick call to my mother to tell her what was happening. Then I hurried to pack a suitcase and tried to think of all the things I needed to do to have things in order for Joe and Kathy in the event I ended up having to be away from the house for any length of time.

My mind whirled with activity trying to remember everything I should do when I realized I had to call Kathy's school to let them know my aunt would be picking her up because of a family emergency. I knew Kathy was going to be upset by my sudden departure and that I wouldn't be able to personally bid her goodbye.

We checked Kari into the hospital at 3:00. She didn't complain when I readied her for bed. I'm sure it was because the headache and vomiting were making her miserable. Certain doctors were permanently in charge of her case, but there were always others assigned to take care of her. I hadn't met the doctor she had this time, although I did remember seeing him at the clinic.

He did a lumbar puncture and found leukemia cells in her spinal fluid as we feared. One of the drugs had to be injected into her spinal column. Kari was asleep when Joe and I left to drive to Napa. He ate dinner and headed for home on his own with another uncertainty for our little girl hovering between us.

My parents' car was being serviced at a local garage, so I wasn't able to go to the hospital the next day. I called and talked to her doctor. He said she was feeling better, but he'd have to do another lumbar puncture the following day as part of the procedure. I pitied Kari just thinking about the pain.

Mom and I went to a store the next day and bought Valentine cards. I also got Kari a stuffed clown with red hair, dressed in a red and white striped suit. It made a laughing sound when you squeezed its body. I guess it was a little bit of manufactured happiness, but the main thing was it did make Kari smile. She felt well enough for us to have a good visit. The doctor even intimated that she might be able to go home on the weekend.

I dared to feel optimistic, but my spirits were sent plunging down when she started to run another fever that night. The doctor prescribed shots of penicillin. I swear, sometimes it seemed as though that child had become a pincushion.

One of our friends was having complications with a pregnancy and had been sent to the UC hospital at this time. She knew Kari was there and got permission to take her to the playroom where they painted Valentine pictures. It meant a lot to my little girl to see a familiar face. Any pleasant distraction from the disease was always welcomed.

Kari's muscles had begun to react so violently to the shots that the doctor decided to try giving her oral penicillin instead. X-rays were taken of her chest to see if she had some congestion that might be causing her fever. Several doctors were going over her case every day trying to unravel the mystery. The days continued to drag on without any answers.

Joe and Kathy came to Napa for the weekend. Besides having to worry about his daughter, he had his father on his mind. My father-in-law's cancer had put him in the Veterans Hospital in Martinez, California during this time. The hospital was also in the Bay Area, so we took the opportunity to go visit him.

He'd been a plumber for most of his life. The physical labor had fashioned him into a barrel-chested, powerful looking man. His outward nature was quite gruff, but he really was a very tenderhearted man. He couldn't bear to talk about Kari's illness, so we didn't mention that she wasn't doing well.

She continued to burn with high fevers, and one day when I arrived the nurses were wiping her body with cold towels. She whimpered and looked very small sitting there in the big bed. She immediately wanted me to hold her, but I knew I couldn't interfere. I explained the nurses were trying to make her feel better and would be done soon.

I stood in the doorway looking up and down the long hallway as I waited. The scent of illness and medications hung heavily in the air. The ward was filled with seriously ill children. A comatose three-year old girl was sharing Kari's room. She'd fallen off her father's motorcycle without wearing a helmet.

He stood silently by her bed with his hands shoved into the pockets of his jeans. His lips were compressed into a thin, hard line, as he watched her. I can't imagine the weight of the guilt he must have been feeling. The mother sat by the bed. She was pregnant. She kept calling the little girl's name begging her to answer, but the child never responded.

The place was filled with so much suffering it seemed to undulate in waves up and down the corridor. A little boy we'd met from the clinic was across the hall from Kari's room, dying. A two-year girl with her face distorted from a brain tumor was lying on a cot nearby.

The cancer had spread to her spine and she couldn't sit up.

Another young girl, I'd say about eight years old, was wheeling herself down the hallway in a wheelchair. One leg had been amputated because of snakebite. I heard later that she lived in some remote mountain community in northern California and hadn't received proper care soon enough to save her leg.

It was hard not to get depressed in such an environment. I knew good things did happen at this hospital, and some children did go home completely well again. But I saw far too much misery in all the times Kari was confined there.

Our friend gave birth to a premature baby boy three days later, but he only lived for a few hours. I knew how heartbroken she had to be. She'd done everything she could to save her baby, but in the end it wasn't enough. There's a lot of solitude in individual suffering. You find yourself wanting to take on some of that pain to give the sick person a rest from their burden.

It's a wonder after going through so much misery that a person doesn't have certain feelings die inside them. But no one knows how much inner strength they have until they're put to the test. Children are remarkably resilient when it comes to being disillusioned; and Kari was no exception, even though she was being pushed to the limits of her strength.

Joe was very discouraged when I kept telling him the doctors couldn't find the cause of Kari's fever. She was now on an IV because the oral medication hadn't helped. He finally decided to take a day off and come to the hospital. He needed to see his little girl.

My mother bought Kari the book, *Snow White and the Seven Dwarfs*. We took it to the hospital. It ended up being one of her favorite stories along with *Are You My Mother?* I lost count how many times I read those books to her, but she never got tired of hearing the tales.

Joe and Kathy had to go home. I'd been away for two weeks. She wanted me to be home with her. She also missed Kari. It wasn't easy trying to be together as a family.

Sometimes I felt like I was living a double life; one at home and one at the hospital.

Joe and Kathy came back to Napa the following weekend. This time they brought Cuddles with them. Joe said the dog kept going into Kari's bedroom sniffing around. He felt certain she missed Kari and was probably very confused, wondering why she couldn't find her. That little dog had a very strict sense of devotion to our daughter.

We were finally allowed to bring Kari home after three weeks in the hospital – but not before she'd had to suffer through two bone marrow tests, five spinal taps, four injections of drugs, and ten days hooked up to an IV. She was sitting in a wheelchair parked at the end of the hall looking out the big bay window when we arrived. The nurse had surrounded her with pillows because her body was so sore from all her medical procedures.

The doctor who'd been in charge of that particular hospital stay met us there. He seemed as pleased as we were that Kari was finally well enough to go home. He said she would need a lot of rest because she was still weak and tired easily.

Then he got down on his haunches in front of Kari and told her she was a very brave little girl. He looked at us and said she was pretty incredible. I always felt there was something too subtle to define that existed between Kari and the medical staff at UC. He left and we wheeled her back to her room to ready for the trip home.

I had to be very careful dressing her as the slightest movement caused pain. But there was no disguising her joy because she knew when we left this time she would be going with us. She sat on the bed making sure I gathered up all her things she'd accumulated during her stay. One especially nice gift was a clown vase with an arrangement of colorful artificial flowers sent from a couple of mothers from Oroville. The husband of the woman who'd just lost her baby brought it to the hospital on one of his visits.

Kari clearly enjoyed her reunion with Cuddles. It was difficult to say which one was the most excited. The dog usually slept on the floor by Kari's bed, but she obviously had other ideas that night. She was so ecstatic to see her young mistress again she jumped up on the bed and snuggled up close.

Cuddles looked at me with her big, brown eyes as if to say, "I just couldn't help myself."

I let her stay. How could I scold such a demonstration of devotion?

Word had gotten around the clinic among the other parents about Kari's latest hospital stay. Larry's mother heard the news and called us to ask how she was doing. She told me Larry was holding his own but another five year old boy had just died.

Death seemed all too eager to seize its next young victim, as one by one the children we met were being taken away. Sometimes I felt like the leukemia was a wild dog snapping at our heels while we tried to elude the pursuit of the relentless disease. You're running through an unfamiliar forest and you can feel the eyes of the vicious beast watching you.

Kari had to go back to the clinic a week after getting out of the hospital. She had a slight case of tonsillitis, but the doctors were more concerned with her sore ankles. It was especially painful when she tried to walk. Another thing that concerned them was how dangerously close to toxemia she was from the drugs. But they were reluctant to cut back on the dosage because it was keeping the leukemia cells knocked out.

As usual, her treatment was like walking a tightrope without a safety net waiting to catch us if we fell.

Chapter Five

Another week went by without any noticeable improvement with Kari's ankle pain. We took her back to the clinic. The doctors ordered x-rays and decided she probably had calcium deposits. The pain eventually did begin to subside, and Kari was able to place weight on them and run a little. But even better news was having her toxemia finally begin to subside. You could almost hear the collective sigh of relief rippling around the conference room when the doctors revealed the good news to us.

Another small victory over a deadly foe.

We saw Larry's mother at the clinic that day. She said he was in the hospital. I left Kari with Mom and bought a couple of comic books at the newsstand. I went to his room to say hello, but he was asleep. His face had a strained look even in slumber. The healthy flush of youth you'd expect to see in a boy his age was gone.

I couldn't help thinking he should be hanging out with his friends, tossing a baseball around, instead of lying in a hospital bed. I left the books and tiptoed out of the room, hoping he'd soon be feeling well enough to go home.

News came that another two year old boy had just died from his leukemia. Selfishly perhaps, I wished there was some way I could anesthetize myself against the sadness these deaths generated. A person had to learn not to count on having a long term relationship with any of these special children. It must have been unbelievably difficult for the medical staff to endure, since they were so involved in treating all the kids.

Kari did so enjoy her time being at home. Her bedroom became her haven. She'd sit at her little table when it hurt to walk, cutting out paper. She became quite adept with her little scissors and created some pretty unique designs.

She never left a mess with all her paper cutting. I would have picked up a whole ream of paper if I had to just as long as she enjoyed herself. But she was always very neat and scooped every little speck into a wastebasket sitting by her chair.

She learned how to amuse herself because her illness kept her isolated from other kids much of the time. She'd sit there humming or singing and sometimes talking to her dolls in her dollhouse. Making things with her Tinker Toys and looking at the Cinderella book was also favorite ways to pass the time.

It was comforting to see that she could be so content. The boundaries imposed on her life seemed to close in as the disease progressed, but she still managed to sift out a few grains of happiness. I guess I was being unrealistic because I wanted to hold onto the good days, but she was more practical and took what she could get.

Kari may not have been able to play with other children very much, but she did have her faithful Cuddles. They were constant companions. She loved to help me bathe and brush the dog. The little animal would let Kari do just about anything to her, even to dressing her up in doll clothes. Sometimes, if I closed my eyes and listened to her laughter I could almost pretend she wasn't sick at all.

Kathy became very irritable around this time and was having trouble sleeping. She'd burst into tears for no apparent reason and started complaining of stomachaches several times a day. I took her to the pediatrician. He

61

examined her and did some tests, but everything was normal. He suggested she might be suffering from nervousness.

I'd suspected as much. How could she not be upset? Joe and I couldn't completely shelter her from the anxiety that had embedded itself in our family home. Kathy was only six years old, too young to fully understand the full extent of what was going on. But she knew something definitely was very wrong.

She shared a bedroom with Kari. She witnessed her little sister vomiting, heard her cries of pain, saw the endless bottles of medicines, and felt the loneliness during the long hospital stays. The girls couldn't even play together in the same way they used to before Kari had taken ill.

I wrote earlier that Kathy was a timid child. She often displayed signs of insecurity and needed a lot of nurturing. Joe and I did our best to assure her that she was very important to us, even though we had to lavish so much attention on her little sister. I tried to soothe Kathy's fears; but I couldn't shake the feeling that I was neglecting her, and it often weighed heavily on my conscience.

I had to keep relying on family and friends to fill in the void caused by my frequent absences, sometimes on very short notice. Joe's father even did his part by picking her up at school when he was feeling well enough. Joe and I will never be able to thank them enough for all that they did for Kathy. They did the best they could. But they weren't her mommy.

I marveled at how Joe could carry out his many responsibilities as well as he did when his life had to be so terribly distracted. He had his father's cancer to be concerned about besides Kari's ill health. But he couldn't allow his emotions to interfere with his teaching. The wonderful comments his ex-students still make all these years later about him being a wonderful teacher attest to how well he did his job.

I guess I'm just a worrier by nature, and it did bother me that he'd taken on so much in an effort to bring in the extra money we needed. Besides teaching his several high school business classes during the day, which left him with a tremendous amount of papers to correct every evening at home, he was also teaching an adult night bookkeeping class and coaching two sports.

It wasn't just the weight of Kari's illness that laid so heavily on him, but there was also the way that we'd lost so much connectedness in our home life. He had to take up a lot of the parental slack with Kathy when I was away and try to be both father and mother to her.

One special thing Joe did was to take her out to dinner at a local steakhouse one night a week. This was their evening together when he could have the time to focus on Kathy and give her his undivided attention.

We ended March with another trip to the clinic. Kari received a good report. Those were the small moments in time we learned to cherish. Other children didn't fare so well at that time; after hearing that Larry was still in the hospital, I knew that wasn't a good sign.

Once again I went to see him, but he couldn't have visitors. He had pneumonia. I stood there staring at the closed door to his room. Oh God, I prayed, please not Larry. He'd been a symbol of such strength for us all. I thought of all the times he sat with Kari in the playroom at the clinic, drawing pictures with her, or taking her by the hand and walking with her up and down the hallway

when she became restless. I didn't want this to be the end,
unable to accept that the leukemia would win.

Is death the reward for bravery? I silently asked
myself.

I turned away and slowly walked to the elevators –
elevators that would take me back to the clinic and to my
own sick child.

It was getting late as I pushed the down button. A
woman was standing nearby with her back to me, looking
out the window. She couldn't have been seeing much
since it was dark out, but I know what it was like to stare
at nothing. I was just about to step into the elevator car
when she startled me by calling my name.

I immediately spun around. What a surprise to learn
her identity. This was the same woman from my high
school days who'd gathered with the group of nurses at
the Oroville hospital in late 1960 when Kari was ill as a
baby.

I knew something had to be terribly wrong for her
to be there. She proceeded to explain that her eleven week
old baby girl had to have heart surgery. I recognized how
frightened my friend was because I'd been fighting my
own fear for the last year and a half. It's that terrifying
knowledge that tells you what is given so freely can also
just as easily be taken away.

I felt such empathy for her. She looked so
vulnerable standing there by herself. I stepped into the
elevator car and waved to her before the doors slid shut.
It's such a paradox when you're involved with a long
term illness. On the one hand, you're concentrating on
your own problems while at the same time you also
become more cognizant of the suffering of others.

That awareness has deepened over the years for me.
I don't even have to know the people involved, but I still

feel sympathy for them. Depending on your situation, you begin to sift through what you think is doable and what you know you probably can't manage. One thing we'd learned for certain was not to put things off when it concerned Kari.

With that in mind, we decided to take the girls to Disneyland in mid-April 1965. We told Joe's mother and step-father we were heading down their way. It started raining pretty heavily up and down the coast the next few days, and my mother-in-law feared we would cancel our trip. But we were determined not to abandon our plans.

She was so happy to see us that she cried when we walked into the house. She prepared a leg of lamb for dinner and hovered over her two granddaughters, anxious to please. The rain continued all the next day and the children began to get restless. There wasn't much for them to do in their grandmother's small duplex.

I hoped the weather wasn't going to spoil the promised trip to Disneyland for the girls. Thank goodness the rain finally stopped and the sun came out. April 14th is a time that a lot of people probably dread because of the income tax deadline, but it turned out to be a fantastic time for us. Walt Disney really did create a Magic Kingdom capable of generating lots of smiles.

Kari felt well enough to share in all the fun, so we were like any other family with young children enjoying a special day. We rented a stroller, so she wouldn't get too tired. We rode on all kinds of rides. She especially enjoyed the *Jungle Cruise* and *It's a Small World*. We climbed the tree house and zipped around on the Monorail.

Kari shook hands with Goofy, the Three Little Pigs, and Flower, the Skunk from the movie, Bambi. She saw Thumper, the rabbit we all remembered and loved from Bambi; Alice in Wonderland; and Captain Hook. She was absolutely thrilled when the Seven Dwarfs came marching by. It was like having her Snow White book come to life.

I watched Kari's expression, as she stared in awe when the brilliant colors of the fireworks lit up the night sky. I felt more grateful than I could say that we'd been able to share this wonderful day with our children.

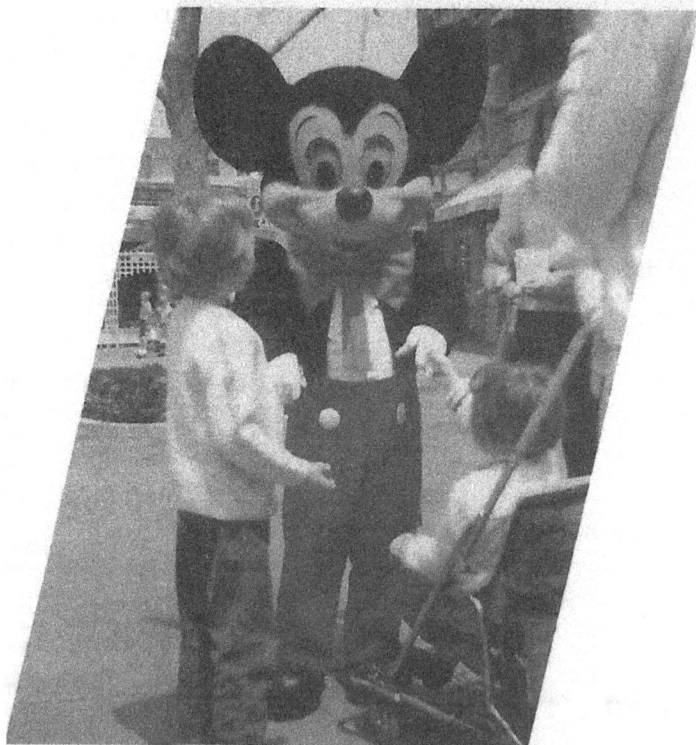

Kathy & Kari loved the Disney characters - 1965.

We had a much nicer Easter that year. I bought the girls matching dresses with white lacy bodices and full canary yellow skirts. My mother bought them each a white straw hat with yellow daisies. It rained that Easter, but that was okay because the girls were our rays of sunshine. We hid colored eggs inside our house, so they could have an Easter Egg hunt before we drove out to the country and a visit with my aunt and uncle.

My aunt took a photo of them standing all smiles in front of her fireplace. It's still one of my favorite childhood pictures of Kathy and Kari after all this time.

Kari had a clinic appointment two days later. Our good fortune continued when her doctors said she was still doing well. We'd go there, they'd do the blood work, and examine her. Then we would sit and wait for the results. It was like pulling the petals off a daisy. Will the news be good, or will the news be bad?

Larry was in the clinic that same day after spending twenty-six days in the hospital. He was on the last available drug to treat the disease, and it had made all his hair fall out. His skin had a pasty look to it and his clothes literally hung on his gaunt frame. He appeared very frail and moved with the gait of an elderly man, rather than the young teen that he was. I felt sick at heart seeing what the leukemia had done to him. I gently touched him on one bony shoulder and said how glad we were that he was out of the hospital.

Kari was so excited to see him that she scrambled onto the chair next to him and started chattering about our Disneyland trip. She didn't see him as being ill. She just knew that this was her friend, and she wanted to share a very happy time with him. Larry sat there smiling and listening to her.

If a person needed to understand the true spirit of courage, they only had to see that young man struggling with his illness that day and how he ignored his pain, so as not to dampen the spirits of his friend.

Larry's mother told me they didn't have insurance, and they were running out of money to pay his medical bills. Her husband was retired and they'd gone through all of their savings. They were going to have to mortgage their house now.

I knew how quickly the bills could pile up because we initially had to get help from my mother-in-law before our medical insurance took over. Even then there are hidden expenses that keep coming to empty your wallet. I urged her to go to the business office and find out if there might be some kind of financial program to help.

As it turned out, she didn't need to go. Larry entered the hospital fifteen days later, hemorrhaging.

He passed away that night.

The social worker saw me at the clinic the next day and sat down to deliver the sad news. I knew this was coming, but the harsh reality of his death left me feeling broken inside with grief.

I had been hoping for a miracle to save him. Perhaps the real marvel is that he would no longer be suffering.

We never told Kari what happened to those children when they died. If she did ask where they were, we'd tell her that their clinic days were different from hers. I knew she would miss seeing Larry above all the others.

But maybe she understood more than we realized.

Three days before Larry died, something quite profound occurred. Joe and Kathy were both in school. I was on the couch knitting and Kari was sitting in a nearby chair looking out the window. She had been very quiet and pensive all morning. I kept sneaking little peeks at her wondering if she was starting to feel ill when she suddenly turned to me.

"I'm going to die and go to Heaven, Mommy."

I was so shocked by her words I dropped my knitting. Joe and I had never told her that she had an incurable illness or talked about an afterlife. I wondered where she'd gotten such an idea. I stammered that I loved her too much and would miss her.

She looked at me with such patience, as though I was a child.

"I know, Mommy, but Jesus needs me."

She shouldn't be talking about dying. She was only four years old!

"We need you, too."

"Jesus needs me more," she replied in a grave voice.

I couldn't believe we were having this conversation and began to plead with her.

"Please don't go for a long time, Kari."

I was fighting to choke back my tears by this time.

"Soon, Mommy, soon. Heaven is a nice place and Jesus needs me," she repeated.

Then she calmly turned back to looking out the window while I sat on the couch in a daze. What struck me as so amazing was not only her words, but the fact that Kari didn't seem to be a bit afraid by the pronouncement. I waited to see if she would say anything else, but she seemed almost unaware of me now. I continued to sit there going over and over her words in my mind.

What had just happened? Did God speak to my child? I looked around. Was He even now in the room? If so, why wasn't I feeling His presence? Then I recalled my dream about seeing Kari in a coffin. Had that been His way of warning me for what was to come?

Was Kari actually trying to prepare me for her death? I didn't know whether to be grateful or terrified. I was still upset over Larry dying and now I had Kari's unbelievable announcement. I loved my child and this time restraint that had been put on her life by the leukemia made me feel like I was being forced to cram that love into a container that was too small.

She said she was going to die soon. How soon? What did such a young child understand about time? Soon might be tomorrow or perhaps next week, next month, or even next year.

Would I wake up one morning and find her dead in her bed?

Kari's left thigh started hurting. Then the pain moved to her legs, her shoulders, and her back. It got so bad she began to scream. We ended up having to take her to UC. She was taking ten pills a day now, and the doctors decided to try another combination. They were finally able to control her suffering enough for us to bring her home after spending six days in the hospital.

Kari would be old enough for kindergarten in the fall. I was trying to be positive and registered her. She wanted so badly to go to school, but now I wondered if she'd be well enough.

I received a letter from Larry's mother telling me about his funeral. I couldn't help crying when I read it. She also wrote to my mother and said she hoped God would give us the strength we needed when Kari's time came.

This latest combination of drugs gave her a tremendous appetite. Her stomach became very bloated from all the extra calories she was taking in. The added weight put a strain on her hips, and she dragged her left foot when she walked.

Her gait became so ungainly that she starting falling. One day she fell in our living room and hit a magazine rack. It left her with a large, vivid bruise on a cheek. Another fall happened in our driveway, blackening her top lip. Kari wanted to be independent, but I felt like I should wrap her in cotton to protect her.

I wasn't feeling well in mid June for Kari's next clinic appointment, so Joe ended up taking her. The report that day was cautiously optimistic. He stopped at The Nut Tree restaurant on the drive home. This was one of her favorite places. We always tried to go there after her clinic appointments if she felt well enough.

One of the big reasons she liked the place so much was because they had a wonderful toy store behind the restaurant and a little passenger train. Kari absolutely loved riding that train. We'd go inside the toy store and let her pay the twenty-five cents for the ticket.

She was often the only passenger. The elderly man who drove the train dressed in an engineer's hat and bib overalls. He'd make a big display about punching her ticket and looking at his pocket watch.

Then he'd wink at her.

"All aboard!" he'd yell.

The route was always the same, skirting the grounds that surrounded the restaurant, chugging by beautifully tended flower gardens, and well kept orchards. It made me think of Disneyland. You would have thought she was going on a long, wondrous journey by the look on her face. She rode that train many times and enjoyed every ride as if it was her first. It had become a small spark of joy in her life.

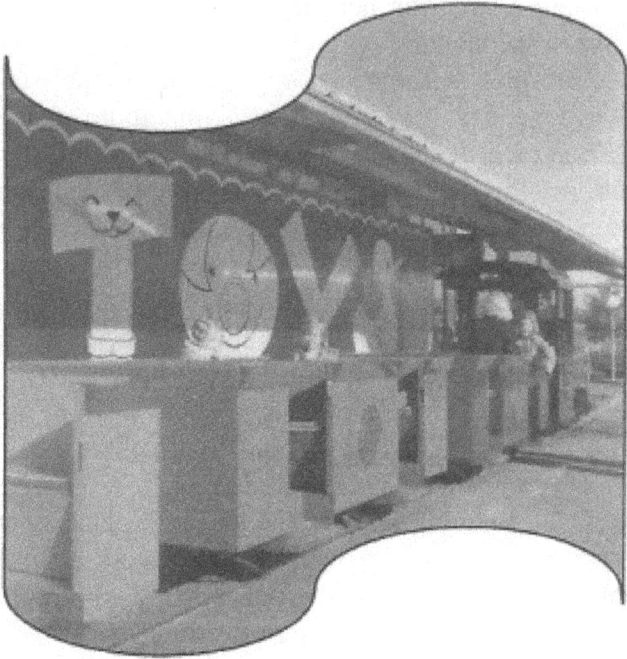

Kari enjoying her favorite pastime ~ a ride on the toy train

We would take her to the bakery inside the restaurant after the train ride. Kari liked to pick out miniature loaves of freshly baked bread to take home. Then, as an extra treat, we'd let her go to the candy section and pick out goodies for the family. She'd walk back to the car, happily clutching her bags of treats.

Another ritual Kari enjoyed on our drives back home was seeing a huge water fountain in the middle of a manmade lake just as we'd leave Marysville. It was the most exciting for her at night because that's when colored lights would come on to illuminate the tall sprays of water shooting into the air.

It was mid-June now, and Joe had started teaching summer school. He was also busy preparing the outside of the house to be painted. Besides that, we have a very large yard for him to take care of. It seemed as though he rarely ever had any free time to just lounge around.

I drove to Napa by myself this time for Kari's next clinic visit. Mom and I took the girls to see the movie, *Cinderella*. Kari was able to follow the plot because we'd read the story to her so many times.

The day ended on a cheerful note, and I tucked two very happy little girls into bed that night.

Sad to say, but that bit of joy was short lived.

Chapter Six

Kari awoke the next morning vomiting and complaining of a stiff neck and headache. This was what I meant when I said we never knew when the leukemia would strike. It rose up once again in a matter of a few hours to spoil what I thought was going to be a good day for Kari.

Mom drove us to the clinic for the scheduled appointment. We didn't need to talk about Kari's latest condition. We'd been through this enough to know these symptoms weren't good, but it's still difficult to completely prepare yourself for the bad stuff.

I received the depressing news that Kari was out of remission once again. Her doctors had no choice but to start her on another drug. The grim reality was that this would be the fourth one, which meant there was only one left of the five to use to treat the disease.

We were surprised to see Larry's mother at the clinic that day. She explained she was there to get the results of his autopsy. I felt ill hearing her say that word. Our visit was bittersweet. I kept thinking about all the times Larry used to walk up and politely greet me.

Something else happened at the clinic that day to add another level of anxiety, as if it wasn't bad enough that I'd been given such bad news about Kari. I saw a woman I'd met a year earlier. Her little boy had passed away from his leukemia and now she was back with another child who'd been diagnosed with the same disease! The possibility that something like that could happen in the same family hadn't occurred to me.

It was June 22 and our eighth wedding anniversary the day I was at the clinic. But Joe and I didn't feel like celebrating, even if we had been able to be together. Kathy's seventh birthday was two days later. I did manage to get her home in time to have a little party. Kari cried when she saw the new bathing suit I bought for her sister because she wanted one, too.

Mom and I took Kari back for her next clinic appointment on June 29th. One of the head hematologists examined her himself this time. He was very concerned about the difficulty Kari was having in walking. X-rays were ordered to be taken on the next visit. He told me the drug she was on now made the bones weak, so he prescribed fluoride tablets. It became another bottle of pills to add to our collection. I'm sure part of the reason she had trouble walking had to do with how heavy she was from the latest round of drugs. Once again I had to buy her new clothes in a larger size because of her increasing weight gain.

Kari awoke on July 3rd with her top lip very swollen and a slight fever. She also had a large blood blister just below one nostril that was very sore because she kept picking at it. Her back was bothering her and she actually asked to go to bed early that night.

She woke up the next morning crying. The back pain had become more intense. I gave her the pain medication the doctors had prescribed and thank goodness it helped. Kari didn't want to do much and spent most of the day on the couch, but at least she didn't complain of hurting.

It was July 4th and we could hear fireworks going off all over the neighborhood. Joe bought a few sparklers and took them outside on our driveway to light them for

Kathy, but they frightened her. My parents happened to be at our house and spent the night.

We were all in bed by 11:00. Kari woke me at 11:45 crying with another backache. I gave her a pain pill and sat with her until she fell asleep again, but she called to me a little over an hour later. I went into her bedroom. I could see by the nightlight that a thin trail of blood was trickling out of one nostril.

I tried everything I could think of, but I couldn't get it to stop. I called our local doctor and told him what was happening.

"Oh yes, this is the little girl with the problem," he said and told me to pinch her nose for five minutes.

It didn't work. I called our hospital next and told the doctor I talked to there that Kari had acute leukemia and had a nosebleed. He advised me to do the pinching nose thing.

Kari was still bleeding after an hour. She wasn't hemorrhaging, but the blood flow wasn't stopping, either. I phoned the pediatric ward at UC in the hopes I might be able to talk to one of her many doctors there, but was referred to their emergency room. A doctor on call took all the information, plus her pediatrician's phone number in Marysville, and said he'd get back to me.

He called a short time later and instructed me to take Kari to the hospital in Marysville where her doctor would meet us. Joe and I quickly dressed. I put a clean nightgown on Kari and wrapped her in a sheet. He carried her to the car while I grabbed her pillow and gave Kathy a quick kiss. She was clearly upset, but at least she didn't cry.

Our one stroke of good luck was having my parents be there with Kathy. I would have hated to call other family members or friends at 4:00 in the morning.

There was only a small smattering of vehicles on the narrow strip of highway that early in the morning. I made Kari a bed in the backseat of the car and sat with her. She was very pale and still bleeding by the time we finished the forty-five minute drive.

The pediatrician examined her and ordered blood work. Kari was too tired to offer more than a few sleepy whimpers. I was relieved to see that her nosebleed had finally stopped. I hoped that meant everything would be all right and we could go back home now.

The doctor returned a short time later with the results of Kari's blood work. He was very sorry to have to tell us that we were going to have to take her to San Francisco. He'd already called and told them to expect us. I wrapped her in the sheet again and Joe carried her out to our station wagon. We readied ourselves for the three hour drive just as the sun peeked over the horizon.

One of Kari's doctors met us as soon as we arrived at the pediatric ward and began treating her right away. He told us he was worried she may have an infection in her blood. He put her on intravenous antibiotics. We stayed with Kari until late that afternoon before driving to Napa for some much needed sleep. My parents had driven home in the meantime with Kathy.

Joe and I visited Kari the next day, and she looked surprisingly well. She was listening to records, but soon asked us to read to her. The doctor put her on a liquid diet. I thought she'd be unhappy about that because she'd been eating so much, but oddly enough her ravenous appetite was gone. Perhaps it was just as well because the doctors were going to try another combination of drugs and take her off the one that had caused her to gain so much weight.

Joe had to drive back to Oroville to teach his summer school classes. Kathy and I stayed in Napa. She stayed with a neighbor while Mom and I went to the hospital each day. The social worker we knew so well from the clinic often came to read stories to Kari. I took along small gifts, trying to keep her spirits up.

Kari's body grew warmer, and her face flushed as her temperature continued to spike; obviously, she was pretty uncomfortable during most of our visits. She kept asking the nurses to take out the IV. Who could blame her? Kari had had enough of them to wish them away. Unfortunately, she had to receive her meds intravenously because her fever persisted.

Joe came on the weekends to see Kari, but she wasn't very responsive. She was becoming very depressed and was barely eating at all, despite the doctor ordering daily milkshakes for her. Besides her fever, he was concerned about a collection of bright red spots that suddenly appeared dotting one cheek, her side, and one shoulder.

Her anemia was very bad and she had to be given blood transfusions and platelets. All the extra weight she'd gained quickly melted away. She was starting to take on a hollow-eyed, emaciated look. Kari barely acknowledged us when we visited her, but would cry when we left.

I spent hours reading to her and playing *Puff the Magic Dragon* and other songs on the record player. Although she always enjoyed stories and music, none of what I was doing could even bring a smile. There weren't any televisions in the rooms unless a person paid extra for one. I asked the doctor if we could arrange to have one set up for Kari.

He agreed right away. Like us, he was willing to try anything to pull her out of her depression. It turned out to be a good idea, as the TV did help to cheer her up quite a bit. She also wasn't so upset when we had to leave her after each visit.

Kari's hand became so swollen from the IV the doctor had to move it to her foot. She was able to stop the antibiotics when her fever was finally gone. But she did have to have another bone marrow. More needles, more pokes, more pain.

Joe and I asked the doctor on one of our visits if we could take Kari out of her room for a while. We thought a change of scenery might do her good, even if it was just down the hall. He gave us permission to put her in a wheelchair and wheel her down the hallway to the big window there. I knew she liked looking outside. The sun felt pleasant coming through the heavy glass.

Kari wanted me to hold her, so Joe gently lifted her out of the wheelchair and put her on my lap. She was very weak and leaned against me with her head on my chest. She fell asleep almost immediately. I carefully cradled her sick little body within the folds of the blanket, just as I had done that first night when I held her after her birth. I'd had such hopes for my baby girl then. But now I think I knew that any promise for a happy future was gradually slipping away.

Kari was starting to improve little by little, but she was still terribly weak. She wanted me to help her use the bathroom when I was with her, instead of making her use the bedpan. She also liked to eat at the small table in her room when I was there to visit, but it didn't take long before sitting up in a chair would make her tremble from fatigue.

The day finally came when we were able to bring her home again. This hospital stay had lasted twenty-two days. That's a long time for anyone to be away from everything they enjoy, especially for a child.

Home was a larger, older home now, giving the girls each their own bedrooms for the first time. We moved the last day of July, which happened to be my twenty-sixth birthday. We were too busy trying to get settled to do any kind of celebration. I didn't care about having anyone fuss over my birthday, but a friend who was now our new neighbor gave me a smiling white ceramic Buddha figurine. She told me rubbing its belly would bring good luck.

If only!

Kari vomited the very first night in our new home and woke up with her back hurting. I wondered if the move had been too much excitement for her. She did feel better the next day, but that didn't last. She woke me on August 2nd at 4:30 in the morning with a headache and gagging. I gave her a pain pill, and bless that sweet child, she told me I could go back to bed. But I stayed sitting by her bed.

She'd only been asleep for a short time when she woke up again. She said she wanted to see her daddy. I called to Joe and he came into the bedroom. Usually when we'd ask how she was doing, Kari would say, "Pretty good."

But not this time.

"Not good," she whispered.

My heart sank. Our telephone hadn't been connected yet, and there weren't any cell phones back then. I was so thankful that our friends lived just two houses away.

The first blush of dawn was just beginning to color the morning sky, as I stepped outside. I sprinted across our front lawn and the next door neighbor's yard. The grass was slick with morning dew and wet my toes through my sandals.

My call to one of Kari's doctors in San Francisco brought a recommendation to take her to the doctor in Marysville, because of the distance we'd have to drive to get to UC. A short time later, after her pediatrician examined her, he said we needed to take her to San Francisco after all.

Talk about déjà vu.

We got back into the car, and Joe started driving. I felt so sorry for Kari, as she'd just left the hospital six days before. She was asleep on the backseat. I kept turning around looking at her every few minutes. We were about a half hour from the hospital when I noticed her eyes were open, but they appeared glassy and unfocused.

Her face and hands began to twitch. I talked to her, but she didn't respond. Then her eyes started darting wildly about. I told Joe something was terribly wrong and climbed over the seat to be near Kari. I yelled to him that we had to get her to the hospital as quickly as possible. The poor man wove frantically in and out of traffic, doing the best he could, to get us there.

We drove directly to the UC emergency room. Kari was having trouble breathing by then, and her skin had taken on a bluish tint. I grabbed her into my arms and barely gave Joe time to stop the car before propelling myself out of the backseat. I ran into the hospital and quickly told the person at the desk Kari's name and that she had leukemia. After taking a brief look at her, the staff immediately whisked her away.

Joe parked the car and hurried inside. We were sent to a waiting area where we sat on hard wooden chairs in a crowded narrow hall. Children were crying and people were moaning. Some people glanced our way, but most were too distracted by their own problems and ignored us.

The waiting was endless and seemed more like hours. Once again I kept thinking this couldn't be happening, not realizing I was clenching my teeth until my jaw began to ache. I had to grip my hands together in my lap to keep them from shaking.

One of Kari's doctor's finally came to see us. He said this was the worst she'd ever been, and he didn't think she was going to pull through. She was going to be moved to the pediatric ward, but he took us to see her first. She lay on a gurney in a tiny cubicle. She was so still and pale I thought this would be the last time we'd see her alive.

We stayed for hours until the doctor urged us to go and get some rest. He promised to call us if there was any change in her condition. We kissed Kari goodbye and drove to Napa. Despite feeling emotionally and physically exhausted, it was difficult to sleep, but we finally managed to doze off. The shrill ringing of the phone woke us up early the next morning. We rushed to answer it, fearing to hear terrible news, but it was just some young kids playing a prank. Their playful laughter was cruel given our dreadful situation.

Kari had been put in isolation when we went back to the hospital. We had to don hospital gowns and face masks before we could see her. She was finally awake. I saw that she had an IV attached to one foot. Joe and I stood on either side of her bed holding her hands and talking to her. I touched her on one cheek.

She stared at me and asked if I was the lady who . . .

Her voice trailed off before she could finish the sentence. She thought Joe was the man who brought candles. We looked at each other feeling totally confused. She wasn't making any sense.

We questioned her further before we gradually began to realize something was very wrong.

I looked at Joe. The anguish in his eyes matched my own.

"Oh God, I don't think she knows us," I whispered.

Chapter Seven

The doctors had been so busy concentrating on Kari's physical condition they didn't notice her mental state. Although we hadn't lost her in the physical sense, she was for all intensive purposes not our little girl. The leukemia had taken over her brain.

I had another vivid dream that night. All the children we met who had died were coming down the hospital hallway. They were doing the Bunny Hop. It's a kind of dance where you form a single line, holding onto the person's waist in front of you. Everyone kicks their legs out to the right, and then to the left a couple of times before hopping forward once, backwards once, and then forward three times.

They were all laughing and looked wonderfully healthy. The children who hadn't yet succumbed to the disease were standing in the doorway of their hospital rooms. The dancing line stopped at each door and one by one the individual child was asked to come along.

They came to Kari's room and asked her to join them.

"Not yet," she replied.

I told Joe about the dream as soon as I awoke the next morning. He was stunned.

"How do you do that?"

"I have no idea," I told him.

I didn't believe I was doing this to myself. Was this another clue to what would happen with Kari? If she continued to live, would her mental state improve, or would we still be strangers to her?

She showed no signs of improvement after a week. The doctors asked our permission to do radiation treatments on her brain. They explained that sometimes this kind of mental confusion happens in cases like Kari's. Every visit brought a new heartbreak. One day we arrived to see Kari and saw that the lady in charge of the playroom was with her. We watched as the woman held a chain of colorful plastic pop beads in front of Kari's face, trying to get some kind of response. It came as a shock to all of us we when realized Kari couldn't see. I waved my hand in front of her eyes, but she didn't even blink.

Then to further add to our sadness, the next day it appeared Kari had lost her sense of hearing. Joe and I watched helplessly as our child slowly slipped away from us, bit by bit.

Thankfully, she did gradually regain her ability to see and hear. But she'd stopped talking with the exception of one occasion when Joe asked her about Cuddles. Kari said Cuddles was her dog.

She didn't talk. She couldn't walk, and she wasn't responding to anyone. She regressed back to infancy and had to be put in diapers. Her hands had to be tied to the sides of the bed because she kept reaching into her diaper and eating her feces. The leukemia had taken over her mind and altered her looks so much we could barely recognize her as our child. Now the disease wouldn't even allow her a shred of dignity.

Joe and I drove home in between visits to get more clothes and run some necessary errands. Kathy wanted to know when her sister would be coming home. The only thing I could say was that I hoped it would be soon. We went back to the hospital with that thought on our minds.

We taught Kari to kiss us on the cheek and Joe showed her how to give us a hug for Kathy. She obeyed like a little robot. Otherwise, she'd just stare into space, slacked jaw, and without a hint of recognition for anyone or anything. It was as though she was burrowed into a dark tunnel so deep, no one could reach her.

Her doctors decided to let us take her home after she'd spent nineteen days in the hospital. They hoped being in familiar surroundings might help her regain her memory and begin to react to us in a positive way. It seemed like a logical thing to do since nothing they tried had done her any good.

I placed Kari's Virgin Mary statue in her hands that first night at home when we put her to bed. Joe and I watched as she clutched the statue in her hands. And then, in a slow, halting voice she began to say her little prayer. What an amazing breakthrough. We couldn't hold back our tears.

It brought to my mind the day Kari talked about Jesus. Now her first words just happened to be a prayer. How could I not believe something very special was taking place?

Joe's belief in God had been badly shaken since Kari's illness. He began to question the teachings of his faith. He had trouble accepting why God would allow something so terrible to happen to our child.

I didn't know what to think most of the time during those awful days, but I prayed for guidance. I kept trying to understand why this terrible thing was happening to Kari. I couldn't find one convincing reason to justify the heartache we were going through, as we watched our child suffer. I felt like I didn't have any power over anything. The leukemia took precedence over all, often undermining what little confidence I tried to maintain.

Joe's father and step-mother wanted to come and see Kari soon after we brought her home from this last hospital stay. We did our best to try and prepare them ahead of time by explaining that her mind wasn't the way it should be. They walked into her bedroom and kissed her. She didn't respond to anything they said or did. My father-in-law gave up after a few more minutes. He gave Kari a couple of awkward pats on her hand and left the room, but not before I saw tears running down his cheeks.

I was changing Kari's diaper in the living room. She'd been home from the hospital for four days and still didn't recognize us. She suddenly began to cry and I thought I might have stuck her with a pin. The crying surprised me because she hadn't uttered another sound since that first night after saying her Virgin Mary prayer. I tried to comfort her, but she kept crying in soft, piteous sobs. I sat on the floor rocking her in my arms feeling so sad for her I ached.

"Are you hurting somewhere, Kari? Tell Mommy," I pleaded.

"I want my mommy," she wailed in a raspy sounding voice.

My heart began to race with excitement. All I could think of was that she was talking and she wanted me. I told her I was her mommy, but she didn't seem to understand. I wished more than anything that I could rescue her from her terrible isolation.

I kept talking to her hoping the veil of confusion would lift from her muddled brain. If we couldn't get through to her she would be left to battle her illness alone without realizing she had a family who loved her. I felt so heartbroken I couldn't even find the words to pray anymore.

She stopped crying as suddenly as she began. I looked at her, and she stared back with more interest in her eyes than she'd shown in weeks.

"Mommy?"

"Yes, sweetheart, I'm your mommy."

Kari gave me a big, beautiful smile and nestled against me.

"Mommy!"

I felt like laughing and crying at the same time. I held her close savoring the hug she gave me in return. I called to Joe and Kathy. They both came running into the living room and stopped. Kari looked at them and said their names. Pretty soon we were all sitting on the floor and hugging each other.

It was the breakthrough we'd been hoping for, although it took another nine months before Kari regained her memory completely. At first she couldn't say her letters or numbers, and when she wrote her name it came out scrambled. I would recite nursery rhymes to her and deliberately put in a wrong word.

"Little Miss Muffet sat on a tuffet, eating her curds and whey. Along came a cat . . ."

Kari would shake her head. "Not a cat. A spider," she'd correct in a grave little voice.

She went through different personality changes during this time. Sometimes she'd be very serious and hardly talk at all. Then the pendulum would swing the other way and she was full of laughter and chatter. Sometimes she acted mean, which was a side of her we'd never seen before. I didn't realize a child so young could have such mood swings. I attributed it all to what the leukemia had done to her brain.

Kari was very disoriented in our house probably because she'd only been there two days before the disease messed with her head. She kept crying and telling us she wanted to go home. We tried to explain to her that this was her home, but she couldn't understand.

We called the young couple who now lived in our previous home and told them our situation. Would they allow us to bring Kari back to her old house and let her see it, especially her old bedroom?

They agreed, and Joe carried her through each room while I trailed behind them. This did the trick, and she finally did accept our present house as the place where she would be living.

Kari's body was extremely bloated, while her arms and legs were thin as sticks. Her spindly legs made it difficult for her to walk. Shoes hurt her feet, so she wore socks and soft moccasins when she did try to take a few steps. Otherwise, she'd sit with her feet bare. She had this funny quirk about wanting to wear mittens sometimes, even though it was summertime and quite hot.

Most of her rich, chestnut colored hair had fallen out. The few strands that remained had a dingy, gray look about them. Her face was also bloated. She did finally slim down, but her hair never was the same when it grew back. The texture was quite fine and looked like she had chopped at it with her little scissors.

She enjoyed sitting on the front porch in a little round rattan chair. We lived on a busy road and she liked watching all the cars going up and down the street. When anyone who knew us drove by, they would honk and wave at her. She loved the attention that gave her.

Cuddles remained at her side, always there on the porch staying close to Kari's chair.

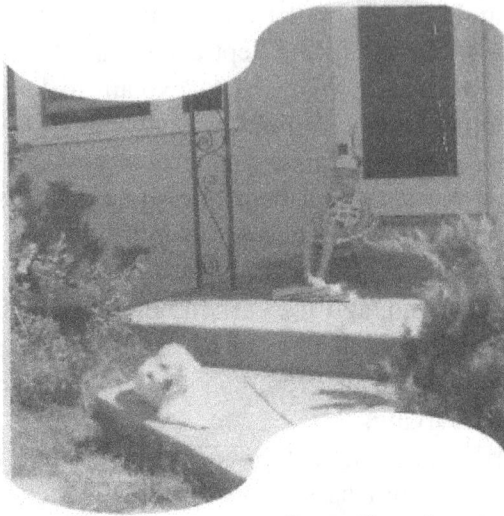

Cuddles on front steps watching traffic with Kari

We took Kari to the hospital on one of her clinic days in September, as the nurses had been asking about her. They were thrilled when she recognized them. That made us all feel good. But the visit was tinged with sadness when we found out another little boy we knew had just died. That meant only Kari and one other girl were left from the original group that had started their treatment at the clinic around the same time.

We gave Kari a small family birthday party in October. She was five years old and had been ill for two years. She enjoyed her gifts and the celebration despite how doggedly the leukemia retained its parasitical hold on her. She started vomiting several times a day for the next three months.

She couldn't stop gagging and was often sitting on the floor in the bathroom holding her head over the toilet. I had to keep a big can by her bed and carry one in the car. Her doctors tried to stop the gagging and vomiting, but nothing worked to reduce it. Kari couldn't sleep through the night because of the persistent retching. I'd hear her and go to her room, but there was little I could do except sit by the bed until the gagging stopped. She developed dark looking smudges beneath her eyes that accentuated her tiredness.

November started with a shaky report at the clinic, followed by another visit and a bone marrow. The doctors were doing everything they could to keep her on the fourth drug. We found out the other girl who had survived as long as Kari died that month. This meant that Kari was the only *old timer* left.

I thought our daughter deserved a badge of courage for surviving such a depth of suffering. I'm not a violent person, but thinking about all the misery she'd been through made me want to smash my fist in the face of the disease.

My family had another valid reason for feeling anxious during that time. My youngest brother, Rodger was in the Marines and fighting in Vietnam. We didn't have the electronics of today to keep in touch with him. He was cut off from us, severed by war in a hostile land half a world away, and we feared constantly for his safety. He did end up being seriously wounded while there.

It upset us to turn on television and watch our soldiers dodging enemy fire and then change a channel to witness people here at home harassing them when they were lucky enough to make it back alive. Rodger was called a baby-killer and had men threaten to beat him up. I realized it was an unpopular war, but why did the people have to take their anger out on our military?

Rodger told us the anti-war demonstrations eroded the men's morale. When a person joins the military, there's always the chance they will have to go to war. That's part of their job, albeit an unpleasant one. There's nothing noble about war; and whatever the reason behind it, people are going to get hurt, and some are going to die.

I wonder how many veterans from Vietnam, some of them still nursing broken bodies and shattered minds feel bitter for the sacrifices they made. Our community chorus and band puts on a patriotic concert every July 4th. During the concert the emcee asks the veterans or anyone currently serving in the military to stand when their service song is played. The Vietnam vets always receive a thunderous applause that goes on for quite a while. I look around the theater, and I can see some of those men actually tremble and tear up.

Kari received a good lab report in December, but she developed a new problem. She became very hyperactive and her body was in continual motion. She kept doing a frenzied tap dance and rattled on incessantly with meaningless chatter. She couldn't seem to stop herself and became wildly reckless.

One time she fell going down the steps to our basement, ending up with a black eye that swelled shut. It wasn't uncommon for her to carry on well into the night until she finally went to sleep through sheer exhaustion. It was a good thing that Kathy had her own bedroom now, so there was more privacy for both girls.

Christmas 1965 arrived, and we were very happy to still have Kari with us. But she couldn't settle down long enough to help much with the preparations that usually gave her such pleasure.

Her attention span was very short, and the frantic busyness continued into February without any sign of letting up. She couldn't seem to control herself as her behavior became more and more erratic. The doctors eventually had to prescribe something to help calm her down.

Maybe I was beginning to appear a bit edgy because the doctors suggested my mother keep Kari for a couple of days while I went home and tried to get some rest.

Mom thought it was a good idea.

But I felt guilty even though Kari was quite happy to stay in Napa. Knowing I wouldn't be much good if I fell apart, I convinced myself this was the right thing to do. But the plan didn't end up working out after all. My mother woke up feeling ill the next morning, and I had to drive back to Napa to bring Kari home.

March blew in cold and windy, while my mother-in-law stormed in with just as much furor.

Unlike my mother, she didn't have the privilege of seeing Kari often enough. The separation helped to feed her anxieties and imagination. She was trying to understand why her grandchild was so gravely ill. She began to form her own explanations.

Was I giving Kari a proper diet? Did I remember to thoroughly wash the insecticides off her fruits and vegetables? She told me I was too young and inexperienced when I'd given birth to the girls.

I needed her support more than her criticism, but I found little solace in self-pity. Although I understood my mother-in-law's distress, I didn't know how to make things easier for her. She was a tiny, high-strung woman with a volatile temper. The pressure of what was happening was very hard on her.

She'd lost her beloved mother to illness when she was sixteen, and her younger brother a year later when he drowned just before his twelfth birthday. Joe always felt those tragedies influenced her for the rest of her life.

I was at Kari's next clinic visit when I saw one of the mothers whose son had recently died. Like Larry's mother, she was there to get the results of the autopsy. She was clearly surprised to see me.

"Is Kari with you?" she asked.

I guess she must have thought Kari had passed away, too. I told her Kari was in the playroom.

She hesitated for a moment.

"Would it be all right if go look at her?" she asked.

I told her I didn't mind. We walked to the playroom together, but I stayed back while she stood in the doorway just out of eye range from Kari.

She silently watched Kari for several seconds before she suddenly walked away without saying another word to me. Maybe she was remembering how her little boy used to play with Kari in that very room.

Kari was very cheerful that day when we met with her doctors in the big conference room. She sang her favorite song, *Puff the Magic Dragon,* to them.

They all clapped making her feel very pleased with herself. These were the brief little pockets of happiness that never seemed to last long enough.

The next morning she felt so ill we had to take her back to the clinic. She had to be hospitalized again. The pediatric ward was full, so she had to spend the first night in the emergency room. The news wasn't good. She was out of remission and had to start the last drug. It had to be given through a vein in three doses, each a week apart. She also had to have a couple of blood transfusions.

This time her hospital stay was another long nineteen days. Kari spent most of the time sleeping, which was just as well because she felt pretty lousy when she was awake. Two days before her release she did feel well enough to leave her room and go to the more pleasant atmosphere of the playroom. She wanted to paint.

She sat before the big easel staining the large sheet of cream colored paper with bold splashes of deep blues, stormy grays, and violent purples. She was smiling, but I suspected the dark colors of paint might have reflected a more somber inner mood.

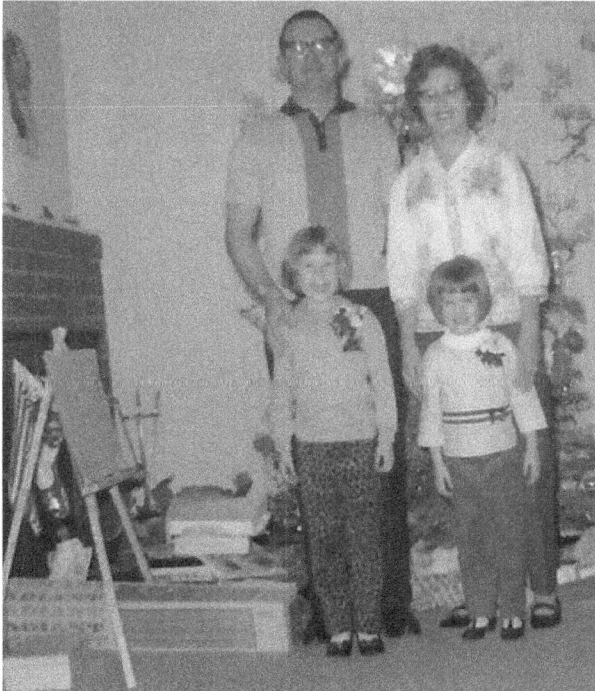

Family Photo taken on Christmas Day, 1964.
One of Kari's gifts was a Painting Easel, standing to the left.
Kari loved to paint at her easel.

Once again, we finally got to bring Kari home. Her hyperactivity had stopped, so she could sit quietly for long periods now. Joe surprised her with a colored television set and had it hooked up ready for use when she arrived. She was still weak from her latest setback, so it was nice to have something she enjoyed to occupy her time while she regained her strength. It also helped to take her mind off the severe stomach cramps she was having from the drug.

Kathy's school was having an open house a couple of days after I arrived home after Kari's latest hospital confinement. Her teacher took me aside and said she was happy to see me back because Kathy had missed me so much. She was like a little building that crumbled every time I went away and had to be rebuilt when I returned.

A new priest came to my church that year. He'd heard about Kari's illness and called to ask if he could come to our house to meet us. She was lying on the couch when he arrived. He told me he had two little girls of his own. He blessed her with the laying on of hands. She stared at him with such a look of serenity I couldn't help wondering who was blessing whom. He had tears in his eyes when he left.

Kari did go back into remission in May. We made weekly visits to the clinic while the doctors adjusted her drug dosage. She seemed to be doing better until she started vomiting again. She also had headaches and ulcers in her mouth.

She ended up in the hospital overnight a couple of weeks later for a blood transfusion and more adjustments to her medications. Kari also had to have another bone morrow done. God, how I hated those things! They always left her so sore she could barely walk afterwards.

We brought her home on our ninth wedding anniversary the end of June. Joe and I were happy to be together for this anniversary, but the best part was having our little girl be out of the hospital once again. Sadly, she didn't feel well enough to help Kathy celebrate her eighth birthday two days later.

Then Kari did start to perk up and feel better. My mother came to our house to take care of the girls while Joe and I went to Reno for a belated anniversary present. I was nervous about leaving Kari, but Mom insisted we needed the time away. If anyone could take care of Kari, my mother was certainly the one. She'd been going with me to the clinic and hospital more than anyone else, including Joe because of his work.

It was a nice idea, but once again the plan fell through. Kari started vomiting and running a high fever while we were gone. Then she started coughing. We finally had a pediatrician in town. The one from Marysville who'd been treating Kari from the beginning of her illness had already made arrangements for this doctor to take over her care in Oroville.

It was comforting to know there was a doctor so close for her now in case Mom had to call for help, but Joe and I decided we needed to get back home. We were nervous that Kari might take a turn for the worse and we didn't want my mother to have to deal with that.

It turned out to be a harrowing trip for another reason. We were driving in the mountains at night and the headlights on our car kept flickering off for several seconds at a time. Talk about scary! We were trying to get home and preferably in one piece.

I have to admit that at times like this I did feel like we were being singled out for more than our share of downright bad luck.

Kari started having more problems with a stiff neck, fever, and vomiting in early July. She had to have a drug injected into her spinal column. Then she began to suffer from intense leg pain. I gave her the pain medication, but it didn't help. I asked for something stronger. She was due to go back to the clinic in four days. I knew enough by now to suspect she would end up in the hospital if her condition didn't improve.

It turned out Kari had pneumonia and was admitted to the hospital. She also needed a blood transfusion. Mom and I went to see her the next day. Kari was in a mist tent. Her color was much better because of the transfusion. We enjoyed a good visit with our little sweetheart.

Kari had to have another lumbar puncture six days later. Then her fever shot up. She was put on intravenous antibiotics and had another blood transfusion. She was so thin her wrists and ankle bones jutted out like little knobs. Bruises were scattered over her body. She actually asked us to leave because she was so tired on that particular visit.

One of the new boys we'd met recently at the clinic was brought into the hospital that night in critical condition. His parents had a priest come to administer last rites. The parents asked Mom and I to come into their son's room to pray with them. I had never witnessed anything like this before, but I couldn't very well refuse. The priest stood on one side of the bed. The parents were on the other side, sobbing as they tried to pray.

I thought how this was the kind of thing I'd only seen in movies. I remember saying to someone years later that I usually avoid watching death scenes in the movies. They told me it was only make believe. Sure it is, but try telling yourself it's no big deal after you've witnessed the real thing.

The boy's room was empty when Mom and I went back to the hospital the next day. We saw the staff washing the plastic that covered the mattress. I didn't have to be a genius to know why.

Chalk up another one up for the monster leukemia.

Chapter Eight

The days passed and brought more misery for Kari. She couldn't urinate, and her stomach became so distended she had to be put on a catheter. She was receiving all her nutrients via an IV now. The doctor tried taking her out of the mist tent; but her fever spiked again, and she had to be put back inside the tent.

Kari was in the hospital for my birthday. She sang the birthday song to me when I told her what day it was. What an incredibly sweet gift from my precious little girl. That she could be so ill and still give of herself in this way touched me more deeply than I could say.

What an exquisite little human being she was. No wonder we loved her so much.

Joe's priest friend was in the area visiting his mother. She and I had been corresponding via letters on a regular basis ever since she sent Kari the Virgin Mary figurine. They came to meet Kari for the first time. They told us later it was a very humbling experience for them. She was able to get out of the mist tent for a little while and sit in a chair. It was nice for Kari to finally meet the woman who'd given her that special statue.

I met some new people at the hospital during this time. One was a husband and wife whose thirteen year old son had leukemia. The other was a woman whose nine year old daughter was suffering from Hodgkin's disease. They took a special liking to Kari and would often stop by her room to say hello. The lady brought her a doll.

We spent quite a bit of time talking together during the long hours we were at the hospital. We all became close, very quickly, clinging to our companionship because so much of life's harmony eluded us in those trying circumstances. Misery loves company, as the saying goes, but in our case I think need was a more appropriate word. Who better could know how we were feeling than someone who was experiencing the same heartache?

The mother of the girl was usually there on her own because her husband's job made it difficult for him to leave home. Her daughter had just spent four months in the hospital and had been home for only one week before she had to return for this latest stay. They lived a long distance away from San Francisco.

It was becoming more and more difficult for the woman to deal with her daughter's illness on her own, and she worried about the younger children she'd left at home in the care of relatives. They missed their mother and wanted her home with them. I knew how that went. The sick one isn't the only child who suffers.

I often saw her in the hallway crying. Mom and I felt so sorry for her. We did our best to offer what comfort we could, but there's really not a lot you can say.

The boy was suffering terribly. He had a fungus infection and pneumonia besides the leukemia. He stopped breathing three times on one of the days Mom and I were at the hospital.

One day we could hear him yelling incoherently. Several nurses ran down the hallway and into his room. He was thrashing about so much they had trouble trying to take care of him.

The day after that I walked by his room and saw a man in there scrubbing the boy's bed. He'd passed away during the night. His parents called me at the hospital to offer support and encouragement. They invited us to dinner later at their home. The mother wanted to show me her son's room and the several bars of soap where he'd carved different crosses. Her husband told her not to talk about it, but it seemed to make her feel better to share her son's unique artwork.

Things were going a little smoother for us, as Kari had started to feel better. Her IV was gone and she was sitting up in bed dressed in a red muumuu instead of the usual hospital gown. I'm glad the nurse who dressed her chose that bright color because she was so pale. She looked hollow-eyed and incredibly frail. I was almost afraid to touch her. This is an awful image to share, but Kari reminded me of the photos I'd seen of people in concentration camps.

She was in the hospital for over a month this time. I was given an armful of medicine when I brought her home. Her stomach was raw inside from the leukemia drug. Other problems started to emerge like greedy wannabes rushing to take advantage of her weakened condition.

She had a fungus infection in her mouth and around her rectum, besides a urinary tract infection. Kari couldn't control her bowels and had to be put back in diapers. All her hair fell out leaving her completely bald. She was getting bloated in her stomach and face like before, distorting her normal appearance once again.

Her legs hurt so much she couldn't walk without pain, but Kari was determined to get moving on her own. She started easing herself out of bed by herself five days after we brought her home. She was very shaky, but she wanted to be independent. She tried to get around by holding onto furniture. One ankle was so sore it barely worked. She moved like an old, arthritic woman weakened by age and painful joints.

When she finally managed to make her way into the living room, she gave me a big smile.

"See, Mommy, I can do it."

I didn't miss the pride in her voice and was glad I hadn't rushed to help her like I'd been tempted to do.

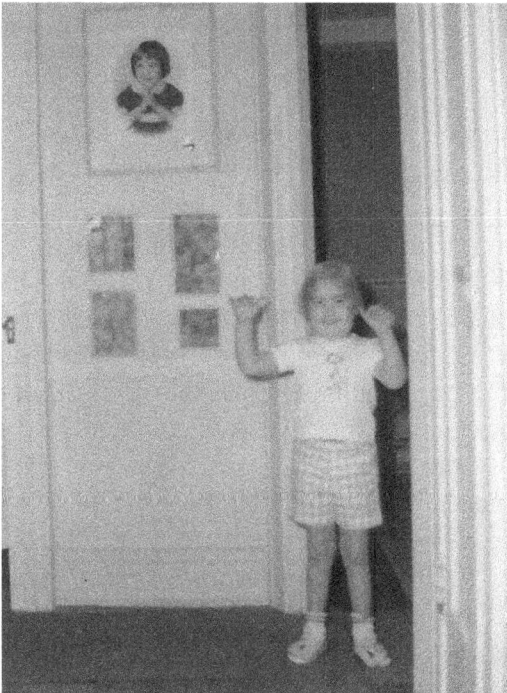

*In September 1965, after being off her feet since July 4th,
Kari shows us she can stand again without falling.
"See, Mommy, I can do it," she said.
She also took pride in showing off her paintings on the wall.*

Joe and I took Kari back to the clinic for a checkup on August 16th. She was only in a partial remission, so the doctors tried yet another combination of drugs. It was a complicated formula that had to be remixed over and over again. They couldn't be sure what would work for her, but they had to keep trying. I always thought the disease had all the deviousness and efficiency of a skilled predator. The trick was for the doctors to be more ingenious than the leukemia.

Kari sang to us all the way home. She'd been making up her own songs for quite a while and they always had to have a title. She liked to sing a few words and ask us to guess what she was going to call each song. If we came up with an idea that suited her, she would smile and tell us we were right.

But I'd often say I didn't know just so she would have to tell me her title. A couple of titles I remember were, *Low High Was A Lady*, and *See There, Daddy*.

My mother came to help us paint the inside of our house. It'd been built in 1929 and owned or rented by several families before we moved there in 1965. The place had been through a lot of wear and tear over the years. It needed a lot of sprucing up, including new carpet and drapes among other things, but we didn't have the money to do everything at once. We bought the house because it had plenty of room, and we were able to get it at such a reasonable price.

Mom and Grant's wife surprised me when I was gone one day and decorated the master bedroom. My brothers, their wives, and my parents helped Joe pay for everything. I loved it!

Kari got a kick out of all this redoing, but she made it quite clear she didn't want us to change her bedroom. I personally thought the red wallpaper and pink painted woodwork from the previous owners was kind of gaudy, but Kari liked the bright colors. Perhaps that was partially true because of all the times she had to stay in the more subdued neutral colors of her hospital rooms.

My Aunt June wrote a letter to the local newspaper around this time telling about Kari and how bravely she was fighting her illness. She mentioned how much Kari loved her little poodle and receiving mail. The response was incredible. People started sending her get well cards. She even received one from Oroville's mayor. She also received all kinds of toy dogs, including a huge box of stuffed animals from the Sheriff's Department.

One day a young girl we didn't know came to our door and gave Kari a small ceramic dog she bought with her own money. Joe and I were very moved by the outpouring of compassion by so many strangers. Their kindness gave Kari hours of happy pleasure. She struggled every day to climb on the couch and watch for the mailman.

A week after her clinic visit, Kari started to have pain in her left arm and hand. I gave her the pain medication, but as usual, it didn't bring her total relief. The pain moved around to different parts of her body and began to intensify. I called one of her main doctors at UC, but he wasn't there. The doctor on call prescribed something stronger. He was kind enough to call me back later and ask how Kari was doing.

Another clinic day was coming up, and I was concerned what it would bring. Would her doctors be able to carve out another narrow escape for our little girl? If not, what could anyone possibly do for her now? Kari was on the last drug. If it wasn't working, there would be nothing else to try. She had to be put in the hospital.

Have you ever had the feeling you were standing on the edge of a cliff with the ground slowly giving way, and you didn't have anything to hang onto?

Joe and I went to see Kari the next day. We were having bright sunshine at home, but San Francisco was shrouded in a mantle of fog. It cloaked the city in a gray mist, robbing everything of color. Our car was sandwiched in among the mass of other vehicles and we crept along like one huge mechanical blob. The dreary surroundings certainly matched our bleak mood.

Kari was in such good spirits when we arrived that I begin to think maybe things weren't so bad and the doctors were just being overly careful by putting her in the hospital. Maybe she just needed a blood transfusion and we would be taking her home soon.

Dream on, Claire, dream on.

Her doctors were not happy. The bone marrow they'd taken earlier showed Kari was having a relapse. Joe and I were just sick at the news. We masked our distress with smiles and read Kari the latest batch of get well cards we'd brought from home. We also gave her a white stuffed poodle from the Sheriff's Department.

Kari was so thrilled I wished the person who'd picked it out could have seen her big grin. It was the nearest thing to Cuddles she could have. She named it, "Little White". They also sent her a pink stuffed elephant with blue satin ears. She called that toy, *Pinky*.

She was still feeling well enough the following day to be out of bed and on the couch in front of the window. The heavy fog from the day before had lifted and shafts of sunlight were streaming into the room. The golden rays gleamed over the dome of her bald head. Joe took her picture, and Kari gave him a big, beautiful smile.

It was the last photo we would ever have of our sweet little girl.

She was wearing the pair of red slippers I had knitted for her the previous Christmas and the Cinderella watch that never ran. Whenever we'd asked her what time it was, she would always say, three o'clock. I bent to kiss her and caught a faint whiff of the cologne my aunt had given her. Kari had always liked girlie things, including getting into my makeup, and wearing my costume jewelry.

Several picture books and records were scattered over the couch cushions. She was holding her new *Little White* and listening to *Puff the Magic Dragon* song on the record player. The nurses checked on her frequently making sure she had plenty of things to keep her entertained. Kari was happy in her own way and I hoped it would last for a while.

Time can be your friend, or it can be your enemy. Either way, it goes on no matter what.

Kari was in bed the next day when we went to visit. She complained of a headache. She vomited, and slept through most of our time with her. The doctors decided to order another bone marrow and have a culture done to see if she would be able to reuse any of her earlier drugs. They warned us that there was only a remote possibility of that, but there's always that spark of hope that keeps you searching for a miracle.

We could see signs of deterioration in Kari's condition on each visit. Her bottom lip became swollen and bleeding. One eye was swollen shut and then the other one closed. She was bleeding from the nose and running a fever. We asked the doctors to keep her as comfortable as possible. No more shots, spinal taps, bone marrows, or transfusions to add to her suffering.

A nurse we hadn't met in any of Kari's earlier hospital stays came in and gave Kari a shot anyway. Our poor little darling cried so piteously it made me want to take on her pain. Joe was so furious he yelled at the woman to read the doctor's instructions.

My parents were in Las Vegas visiting my mom's oldest sister, my Aunt Olivia. They'd planned the trip while Kari was still feeling pretty well. They were very upset when I called and told them what was happening. They said they would drive home the next morning. My aunt asked to come with them.

My father became so depressed and withdrawn when he saw Kari that he wouldn't talk to anyone. Dad was a very prideful man, and he liked to control things as much as possible, but Kari's illness was something he could not bend to his will.

One of Kari's pediatric hematologists came to her room. He had been involved with her case from the very beginning, and I'd met with him many times. He was carrying her medical folder. It was quite thick and frayed at the edges from being handled so much. I recalled how thin it had been that day almost three years before when I was first given Kari's diagnosis.

The doctor turned to the last page. It seemed to me he was taking an awfully long time to study it. I had the impression he was searching for something positive to say. He talked about Kari's latest blood work, which was pretty depressing. I sensed that he was skirting around the real issue.

I finally told him I realized what was happening. He nodded, and then he stared at Kari. He looked so sad I almost felt like I needed to comfort him. He was marvelous with the kids at the clinic, and they all clamored to get his attention. It must have been very difficult for this kind man to watch time and time again and see what the leukemia did to so many of his young patients.

He was a big man with a ready smile and a deep laugh. I usually met with him in the big conference room along with several other doctors at the end of Kari's clinic visits. He was one of her favorite doctors. He would scoop her onto his lap and ask her if she had a song for him. Sometimes she would do a little dance for him if she felt well enough. I remember how he folded his big hand over her restless fingers when she'd gone through that period of being so hyper.

Kari was too weak the next day to talk much. We kept telling her how much we loved her.

"I know," she answered, a couple of times.

She drifted between sleep and awareness. Her body was so bruised she looked like she'd been battered. Her paleness gave her skin a translucent quality. You could easily see the pattern of delicate blue veins at her temples and on the back of her hands.

It was too painful if we held her, so we sat by her bed gently stroking her cheek or hand. She began to gag, so I grabbed a pan and held it to her mouth. She vomited up quite a bit of blood. I don't get squeamish at the sight of blood, but it was frightening seeing so much come out of Kari. I heard her whisper something, as I wiped her mouth and leaned closer to hear her.

"Take care of Cuddles for me," she murmured.

Those were the last words she ever spoke to us.

I read somewhere that you will know when it's time to let a loved one go in circumstances like this. Kari had told me that Jesus needed her. I knew in my heart I had to accept that her earthly life was coming to an end. I knelt by the bed at my parents' house that night and prayed God would take my little girl and free her from her suffering.

She passed away the next morning. It was her daddy's thirty-fifth birthday.

Chapter Nine

We weren't with Kari when she died, much to my everlasting regret. I recalled how I'd stood at the bedside of that boy I'd barely knew while the priest gave him last rites and now I hadn't been there for my own child.

When I talked to Kathy via phone she cried and begged me to come home. She was starting a new school year and wanted me to take her that first day. I'd been like a phantom mother passing in and out of her life for the last three years. I was so torn I didn't know what to do. My mother and aunt offered to drive me to Oroville. I talked to the doctor and he felt Kari could hold on until I returned. I don't know why it was suggested that Dad and Joe stay in Napa rather than the hospital.

I took Kathy to school, met her teacher, and rushed home ready to drive back to San Francisco to see Kari. It wasn't to be. Joe phoned the house while I was gone and said it was over. The hospital had called telling him if he wanted to see Kari one last time he'd better hurry.

He and my dad got there as soon as they could, but she had already slipped away. Joe went into her room and kissed her. He told me later that her body was already cold.

Did Kari know the end was near when she asked us to take care of her dog? I'm still riddled with guilt that we weren't there when Kari breathed her last. It's so upsetting that we had all misjudged her failing strength.

It seems cruel that Kari should have died without having any of her family with her. We'd tried so hard to do what we thought was best for our child throughout her illness, but the leukemia always called the shots.

The disease had been the grand manipulator. All we'd ever done was put up a few temporary barriers. It seems a gross sin against nature that a budding child should die without ever having the opportunity to reach full bloom.

Larry's mother called two days after Kari passed away. I was surprised to hear from her. We hadn't been in contact since her last letter. She told me she'd awakened the night before and saw Kari standing at the foot of her bed. I was stunned. The experience had left her very shaken, and she couldn't understand why it had happened to her. She wanted to know how Kari was doing. When I told her Kari had died, the poor woman broke down and started sobbing.

That strange encounter was just one more mystifying event that had started with my dream about Kari dying in childhood. Larry was the one child Kari had bonded with more than any of the other children she had met at the clinic and hospital. Why had she appeared before his mother instead of me? Had Larry sent her? I doubt that I'll ever know.

I wonder how many other secrets Kari took with her when she died.

We buried Kari in her favorite red dress with the white polka dots. Joe's Lion's Club had given her a small stuffed lamb a few months earlier. She named it, "Lambie" and slept with it when she was home. We buried it with her. The casket was white. We kept it closed. I never saw her in death. I hope I'll be forgiven for not being with her at the end.

Joe and I chose a private graveside service with just family attending. We'd already been through so much we felt it would be easier than a mass in church. We did have a Catholic priest do the burial rites.

The day of Kari's funeral dawned bright and clear, with only a few flimsy clouds that reminded me of torn tissue paper. The sweet aroma of freshly cut grass filled the air around the cemetery. I thought of that lovely fall day when we'd brought Kari home after her birth. Now she would be going to a different home.

The funeral director reached under the flower spray covering the coffin lid and handed me a small gold plated crucifix after the service ended. I have it hanging in one of our spare bedrooms. You think of families being given a folded American flag when a veteran dies as a token of their service to their country. I think of this cross as a token to Kari's courage and suffering. Who better symbolizes those qualities than Jesus himself?

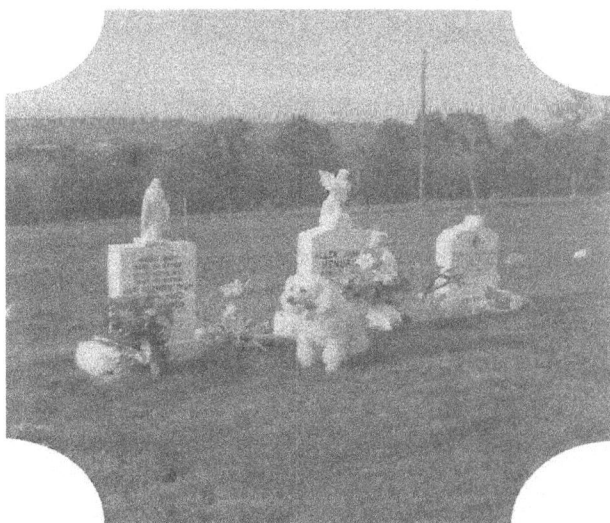

Cuddles keeping watch over Kari's gravesite

Kari's gravesite has a white tombstone with her prayer to the Virgin Mary etched into the stone. We did have a white statue of the Virgin on the top of the stone, but it's been vandalized so many times, we've stopped replacing it.

I found out the first time about this terrible destruction when it appeared in the front page of our local newspaper. The gravestone had actually been dug out of the ground and was lying on its back with the statue nearby broken into pieces. The manager of the cemetery hadn't had a chance to contact us yet, as she and her staff were busy going through the grounds and assessing the damage to several other graves. They soon discovered that most of the vandalism involved gravestones belonging to children.

The people who did this were never apprehended. The cemetery workers found several footprints around the graves indicating several individuals probably took part in the sacrilege. Beer cans, empty liquor bottles, and drug syringes were strewn over the lawn. It made me so angry to think of what those people had done. They were lucky enough to be alive, and there they were partying over the graves of children who never had their chance to live a long life.

Kathy told us a few days after Kari's death that she wanted to move downstairs and sleep in her little sister's bedroom. I was surprised that she'd want to do this, but kind of glad because it wasn't easy walking into that empty room. Well, actually it wasn't empty in the truest sense because Cuddles was sleeping in there. She spent hours every day on the floor next to Kari's bed.

I'm sure she was waiting for her friend to come home like she had so many times before.

It wasn't easy going through Kari's belongings, especially the things that had been with her in the hospital when she died. The funeral home sent someone to San Francisco to collect her belongings. They brought them to our house in a large green bag. I stared at it, knowing that inside were the last things she had touched.

We donated her toys to the Sheriff's Department. Most of the stuffed animals they'd given to Kari were still like new. She hadn't even had a chance to play with most of them. I put them in a large box and sent it to the UC hospital for the pediatric ward playroom. Maybe some other ill children might be given one to cuddle when they were lonely and afraid while being away from their families. My Aunt Olivia had two granddaughters the same age as Kari, so we gave her all of Kari's clothes to take back with her.

Kari enriched our lives with her presence, but she was a precious little gem that we weren't meant to keep. It's very hard not to miss someone you loved so much. You have your memories, but they are not flesh and blood you can hold in your arms. Nor do they give you the sound of their laughter.

Only the cherished echoes remain.

Kathy woke up in the middle of the night calling Kari's name three weeks after she passed away. I hurried into the bedroom and found her crying. She told me she missed Kari. Joe and I had done our best to try and prepare her for her sister's death, but like Cuddles, she was used to seeing Kari leave and eventually come back home again.

I did tell Kathy toward the end of Kari's illness that one day we would not be bringing her home from the hospital because she was sick with something the doctors couldn't make better. I'm not sure if she understood what that really meant.

I think the idea that death takes a person away permanently is a difficult concept for young children to grasp. Forever to them could be as short as a few days. I'm sure there were times when I was away from home for so long that Kathy may have feared I wouldn't be coming back home, either. That could have been part of the reason why she was so apprehensive and usually cried for me to stay with her.

Kari's UC doctors told me that Kathy would take her cue from me, depending on how I reacted after Kari's death. They explained the more emotion I showed, the more upset she would be. I knew I had to try to make the transition as painless as possible. It was going to be difficult enough having to adjust to losing her little sister.

The turmoil Kari's illness caused in our family had clearly been a big strain. I remember seeing a photo of Kathy at a family gathering shortly after Kari died and thinking how sad she looked. Now that I think about it, Joe and I didn't look too perky ourselves.

Kathy tried to do what she could to cheer up her sister, despite being so young herself at the time. She spent hours showing Kari familiar toys and saying nursery rhymes after the leukemia scrambled Kari's thought processes. She has her own special memories of her sister and keeps a few items that belonged to Kari on a display shelf in her home to this day.

My mother and Aunt Olivia went to pick Kathy up at school the day Kari died. The plan was for them to tell her about Kari while I stayed at home trying to compose myself. I was waiting for her in a small room just off the hallway at the side entrance. Kathy stood there silently staring at me. I couldn't tell if she was going to cry or not.

"Are you okay, Mommy?" she finally asked.

I could hear the uncertainty in her voice and knew I had to be strong for her. I pulled a smile out of somewhere.

"Yes honey, I'm okay."

I was grateful my voice didn't betray how broken up I really felt when I saw her relax.

She'd had to cope with the uncertainty of Kari's unstable health. They'd shared the same bedroom for most of Kari's short life and had spent many hours playing together. Kathy was only five years old when Kari was diagnosed with the leukemia; and for the following three years, she rode the roller coaster of her sister's illness right along with us.

At first Kathy said she wanted to go to Kari's funeral, but then changed her mind. Joe and I didn't want to force her. She did ask to go to the cemetery later that day to see the gravesite. The little mound was piled high with flowers. I looked up at the sky, thinking, *we have our own little angel now.*

But then we always did.

I think it really hit me at that moment that our little girl was truly gone. I would never feel her hug me again or hear her tell me she loved me. There would be no more singing or funny jokes. But I also reminded myself there would be no more pain.

I tried not to talk about Kari's illness too much around family and friends, but I suppose I did more than I should have at times. I didn't want to make people feel uncomfortable, but sometimes I just needed to unburden myself. It was my way of releasing the tension that would build up inside me because I was so afraid for Kari.

A couple came to our house right after she died and I poured out all the sad details about her last days. It couldn't have been very pleasant for them, but they'll never know how much their quiet listening helped me to cope with my sorrow.

I don't want to give the impression that I spent the entire three years of Kari's illness constantly complaining. I held a lot of my feelings in and always tried to put up a brave front. People used to tell me how strong I was, but that distinction really belonged to Kari.

My Aunt Olivia invited us to come and spend Christmas in Las Vegas that year. We decided to go. That first holiday without Kari was going to be hard enough. We thought it might be easier for us if we went away from home and the memories of how much she loved Christmas.

It wasn't. We could leave our house, but we couldn't leave our sadness behind.

Although my relatives did their best to entertain us, no one could fill the void we were feeling. When Joe saw one of my aunt's granddaughters wearing Kari's blue coat and matching hat, it was almost more than he could bear. I knew they meant well, but losing our daughter was still too fresh in our minds.

It wasn't easy for Kathy, either. She looked around at all the strangers at the family gift exchange on Christmas Eve. She watched the kids opening their gifts, laughing and talking among themselves, and silently began to cry. One of my adult cousins, whose daughter had received some of Kari's clothes, saw the tears and handed Kathy a present.

"It's okay, honey," she said. "Santa didn't forget you."

That was very sweet of her. But nothing could change the fact that at eight years old, Kathy had lost her sister and her best friend. There aren't enough presents in the world to take the place of losing someone you love.

My father-in-law had to go back into the hospital while we were gone, which made it even more difficult to enjoy the holidays. We stopped to see him on our drive back from Las Vegas. He was very sick. He'd been in the hospital before and always recovered enough to come home, but now he told us he didn't think he was going to make it this time. His stomach was very bloated despite the doctors having drained a lot of fluid. He'd lost a lot of weight and slurred his words because of his weakened condition. I knew death would splinter our family once again.

He passed away a week later.

It'd only been a little over three months since Kari died. He'd fought to stay alive, so he could see his granddaughter until the end. Joe was still struggling with the grief of losing his daughter and now he had to go through it all over again with his father. Like Kari, my father-in-law had battled his illness that had dragged him through the gutters of hell until his strength finally gave out.

He'd told Joe at Kari's funeral that it should have been him. I think he just kind of gave up after she died. He mentioned how much he liked her simple outdoor service. So Joe and his step-mother made arrangements for a graveside service with my priest doing the officiating, as his dad didn't have any church affiliation.

The weather wasn't as pleasant as the day of Kari's service, but this was lackluster January now without the colorful richness of autumn. Damp fog covered our clothes with a misty sheen. We sat together on the canvas chairs the cemetery custodians provided, and stared at the coffin. I couldn't help shivering despite the heavy coat I wore. The leaden sky, shriveled leaves strewed over the ground, and the soggy grass made the surroundings dreary.

I couldn't stop shaking. It wasn't just the cold. I felt the strain of being there. I'd been exposed to too much sadness and death. I sat dry eyed. I didn't have any tears left. I felt depleted and used up. Fragments of happier memories the family had shared seemed distinctly remote.

Joe sat next to me, also dry eyed and stoic. I worried for his peace of mind. He'd lost two special people in a short period of time after watching them both go through terrible suffering. He gave his father his last shave and told me later that his dad told him he'd been a good son.

What is in store for our family now? I wondered. *All the sadness we've gone through makes me afraid to hope for anything.*

The future continued to be stretched out as colorless and murky as the sky, in my mind.

Three months later, the light began to shine from behind the clouds; I discovered I was expecting another child. I can't find enough words to describe how fantastic it felt to have something so happy to look forward to. What better way to heal the brokenness in our family than to have a new baby to join us?

I knew my parents were going to be excited to know that I was expecting again. I wanted to tell them in a special way, so they could share our special joy.

Finally I came up with an idea I thought they would like. I composed the following poem, especially for them, to show my love and gratitude for their continuous support:

Grandparents you are,
Grandparents you'll be.
A boy for Joe
Or a girl for me?

November is the month
Our baby is due.
Start counting the days
Until you meet Little Who.

I wrote the words inside a plain white card and glued a picture of a baby on the front. My dad was so excited he took the card to work and shared it with his colleagues. Many of them had known about Kari's illness and death, so they were genuinely pleased for Dad. Mom was just as excited and couldn't wait to show the poem to friends and neighbors.

We were all going to latch onto this good news and try to put the painful past behind us. It was time to move on and embrace a fresh beginning. It felt so wonderful to share my joy, because with joy comes happiness, the super glue that mends broken hearts.

I wasn't so gullible that I thought we could replace Kari by having another child. It can't be done. She had been her own special person. Her time with us had been far too short, but I had to accept that it was over. I don't want to give the callous impression that Joe and I have dismissed Kari from our minds. Her memory will always hold a special place in our lives.

Our connection with the UC hospital people hadn't quite ended yet. Nine months after Kari passed away, the pediatric hematologist who had come to her room during her last visit wrote to ask if Joe and I would be willing to return for an interview. He also invited some other couples whose children were receiving treatment around the same time.

The letter explained that the hospital psychiatrist was doing a follow-up study on the parents to see how we were coping after our child's death. He hoped to use his findings to help families in the future going through the same experience. We didn't hesitate. We wanted to do anything we could that might ease their ordeal.

We had a good visit at the clinic the day we went back. We saw several of Kari's doctors and even went to the hospital to see some of her nurses. But I couldn't bring myself to go near the room where she had died.

I reminded myself we were there for a good reason and no unexpected sadness would be waiting for us. Many of the staff remembered us and Kari. They gathered around Joe and I offering warm greetings and congratulations when they saw that I was pregnant.

It took over a year and a half before we received a phone call from the social worker at UC in early 1969 regarding our interview. She explained that the results had been written up in a national magazine. A reporter for the Frank McGee Report show on NBC called her from New York after reading the article. He wanted to feature two families on the show and we were chosen to be one of them.

He came to our house with his film crew to tape our part in the show. We sat around the kitchen table while the reporter interviewed us. It made me so happy to be able to publicly relate what a wonderful little girl Kari had been and how courageously she'd fought her illness.

But we didn't get to see the actual show, as things turned out. The reporter couldn't give us an actual date. It ended up being aired while we were out of state on vacation, where the local station didn't carry the program. We called and told the man what had happened, and he was kind enough to send us a copy of the tape.

I couldn't afford a fancy nursery for my first two daughters, but my mother and a friend made it happen. I'm going to indulge myself and brag about it a little bit.

Kathy had moved back upstairs, so Kari's bedroom was now available again. It's tempting to keep a child's room exactly as they left it after they die. I knew Kari was fond of that red wallpaper and pink woodwork, but I also knew that was part of the past I had to let go of, too.

We didn't know if we were going to have a boy or a girl, so we decided not to go with the traditional blue or pink décor. I choose a circus theme. Mom hung the wallpaper with its little figures of circus animals and clowns. My friend made curtains for the two windows using the color aqua from some of the clowns in the wallpaper pattern. We had new furniture with the exception of the bassinet. It was an antique and the focal point of the room.

The wicker was painted white. It had a high hood and sat on a pedestal. My friend wove ribbons among the reeds to match the color of the curtains. She had used the bed for her three sons. I had a rocking chair for the first time. I loved going into the room when it was finished. I'd sit in the chair admiring everything while I anxiously awaited the birth of my child.

I wasn't the only anxious one. Our new baby arrived nine days ahead of schedule, so Joe and I had another October baby, instead of the November date we'd originally planned. This time, I didn't make it to the delivery room and gave birth right in my hospital bed.

I have to say I'm happy I was in the hospital for the birth. I'd been outside raking leaves that afternoon, when I received a call from my doctor's receptionist telling me he wanted to check how I was doing. I had a new doctor for this pregnancy – an obstetrician this time. The call surprised me because I still had several days before my delivery date, and I'd just been to see him three days earlier. But I figured I'd make a quick trip and come right home. I drove myself to his office.

It's a good thing I went. I told the doctor I was feeling just fine. He examined me and said I was also in labor. I couldn't believe it. Once again, I felt I owed a heartfelt apology to all the women who have painfully long labors.

Michelle Leanne arrived on October 30, 1967, just one hour after the doctor ruptured my membrane. I sometimes joke and tell her she made me miss trick or treating that year.

We had another baby girl to love. She reminded me of Kathy with the same wispy blond hair and light eyes. I couldn't wait to get home and start taking care of her. I felt quite well after Michelle's birth. It wasn't just physical. It was an emotional wellbeing, too.

I was given a surprise baby shower. Many good friends came to wish me well and bring lots of wonderful gifts for Michelle. I knew it was their way of showing how happy they were for us.

I had a new nursery and a new baby. But most importantly, this was a new beginning. We'd come out of a long, dark tunnel and into the light. My family certainly needed that.

We'd been so brokenhearted the first Christmas without our Kari the previous year. Now we could look forward to this Christmas because we had our precious Michelle. I remember coming home that Christmas Eve from midnight mass at my church. I stepped into the house, and the first thing I did was peek at Michelle as she slept. I sat there staring at her for a long time.

I knew no gift under the tree could mean as much to me as this baby did.

I should relay that Cuddles was still an important part of our family at this time. She greeted me at the door when I brought Michelle home from the hospital. I held the baby close enough for the dog to have a sniff. She followed me into Kari's old bedroom and watched as I put the baby in the bassinet. Then she plopped down on the floor next to the basket. I guess she decided this little girl was going to need her, too.

We lost that devoted little dog a few years later. She was hit by a car late one night. We didn't realize she'd gotten out of the fenced backyard. Whoever hit her didn't even stop. We rushed her to the veterinarian, but she died the next morning.

I never thought I would cry over the death of an animal, but I really broke down and bawled. I kept thinking of Kari's last words asking us to take care of Cuddles. Losing Cuddles proved to be very hard for Michelle, too. She is a real animal lover and had grown very fond of that sweet little poodle.

Chapter Ten

I continued to concentrate on being a wife and mother up to this point in my life, but that was about to change. Joe started teaching a Business Law class a couple of nights each week at the local junior college in the winter of 1969, in addition to his regular high school classes. He suggested I go with him and take a class.

My first reaction was to reject the idea. I'd been out of high school for twelve years. I told him everyone would be so far ahead of me I'd never be able to keep up. I kept coming up with excuses. I felt incompetent. I was too old. I didn't want to be sitting in a classroom surrounded by a bunch of teenagers.

Joe did manage to talk me into going, despite my reservations. I ended up enrolling in a Child Development class. At least that was a subject I knew something about. I found the experience to be very rewarding. The teacher encouraged me to keep going when that class ended, so I enrolled in two courses the next quarter.

I didn't have any long range plans at the time, but gradually the idea that I might be able to earn a degree began to take shape in my mind. I made an appointment with a counselor. I told him I would have to take most of my classes at night or in summer session because I had young children at home. He told me it was a long haul doing it that way, but he encouraged me to try.

Time went by, and I slowly began to accumulate quite a few units. I went back to the counselor, and he suggested I declare a major. I didn't have a problem with that because deep down, besides wanting to be a mother, I always thought I'd enjoy being an elementary teacher. What can I say? I love children!

I used to gather a lot of the younger kids when I was growing up in San Francisco and play school with them. I set myself up as teacher and no one ever seemed to mind. I taught the others to sing songs and to even read a little. I also enjoyed reciting poetry to them.

The mothers told my mom they thought my impromptu schoolroom was a great idea. They knew their children were safe, having fun, and all the while giving the mommies a chance to have a coffee break.

But despite realizing I now had a definite goal to get a teaching credential, I still thought about having another child. Kathy was nine years older than Michelle and would probably be out of the house leaving us with an only child at home. I'd always kind of hoped I would be able to have three children if at all possible.

Joe wasn't sure if he wanted us to have another child because he would be forty his next birthday. He also worried we would be pushing our luck. What if I did get pregnant again and something ended up going wrong? I admit I wasn't sure if we'd have the strength to cope.

Fate, luck, hope, or whatever you want to call it won out, and I did get pregnant. The baby was due in March, six months before Joe's fortieth birthday, so at least he could say he was still in his thirties. I would be thirty-one. One of our friends told Joe the law of averages was in our favor, and we might have a boy this time. I gained a little more weight with this pregnancy and went past my due date.

I guess my friends thought these were signs I would be having a boy because when they gave me a baby shower they had "John Joseph" written on the cake. John was my father-in-law's name. I did tell Joe shortly before our baby was due that I thought we should pick out a girl's name just in case.

I went to the same obstetrician who delivered Michelle. He told me he was going to be out of town the day the baby was due and wanted to induce my labor. I said I'd take my chances and wait until he returned. I had this thing about letting nature take its course.

I woke up the next morning with back pain, but since it'd been going on the last month, I told Joe to go to school. I always had this kind of lower back pain during all my pregnancies, so that's why it was difficult for me to pinpoint the actual time I began my labor.

I did take the precaution of calling the obstetrician who was taking my doctor's cases and told them what was happening. They advised me to come to the office to be checked. Mom was staying at the house and wanted to drive me, but I told her it was probably just a false alarm.

Boy, was I wrong!

The doctor about exploded when he saw how far along in labor I was and especially when I told him I'd driven myself to his office.

"I sure hope you're preregistered at the hospital," I remember him saying, "because you're not going to have a lot of time to be filling out paperwork."

I assured him I was all set.

He sent me over to the hospital immediately. Fortunately, it was right next door. A nurse met me with a wheelchair and whisked me directly to the delivery room. I asked her to have someone call Joe and my mother. Joe made it to the hospital just before I gave birth, thirty-two minutes after I arrived.

I swear that little baby would have given us a big wink if it had been at all possible, because John Joseph turned out to be Erica Lynn. She had dark hair like Kari, so I'd had two blonde and two brunette children.

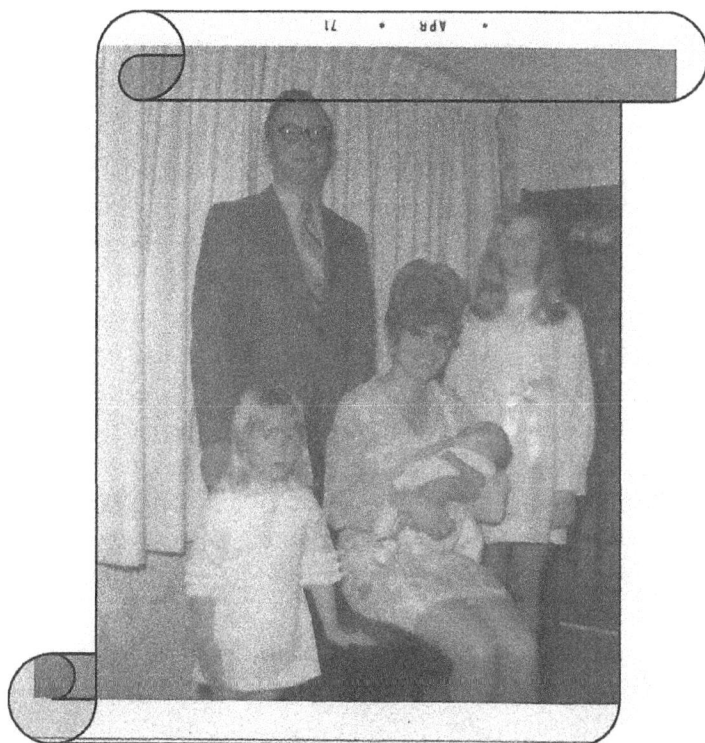

Our New Family: Joe and Kathy in back watching over Michelle and me with new baby, Erica Lynn in my arms.

I mentioned the hair because something kind of cute happened when Erica was very young. She'd been playing outside with Michelle and came marching in the house with a look of fierce determination on her face. She slapped her little hands on her hips and stared at me.

"Am I dopted?" she asked, leaving the "a" off of adopted.

I raised my eyebrows at her.

"No. What makes you think you were adopted?"

"My hair isn't like Kathy and Schelle's."

"Your hair is brown like Daddy's," I pointed out.

"Are you sure I'm not dopted?"

"Would you like to see a picture of me when you were in my tummy?"

"Okay."

I got out the photo album and showed her pictures of me pregnant. I also showed her photos of the day we brought her home from the hospital. That seemed to satisfy her, and she ran outside to play again. I found out years later when we were laughing about this that Michelle had teased Erica and put the idea of her being adopted in her head.

Children are such wonderful, trusting little creatures. That's why we should never abuse their faith in us. It makes me sick whenever I read or hear about someone abusing a child. It's such a privilege when you're given the good fortune to be the guardian of these little souls.

I remember thinking that when 1980 rolled around there wouldn't be any babies for us this decade. Kathy had been born in the 1950's, Kari and Michelle in the 1960's, and Erica in 1971. It certainly wasn't the way I would have planned things, but life is full of too many twists and turns for us to lay out a straight path.

Joe and I feel very lucky that we have three lovely daughters to share our lives. We still think about Kari and wish that she could be here with us. I know in my heart she would have grown into a fine, caring person because the signs were already there, even though she didn't quite make it to her sixth birthday.

I've tried to make sense out of why Kari had to go through such a terrible ordeal, but I don't think I ever will. She didn't live long, but she suffered much too much. I can't help but think of leukemia as a thief. The disease is a robber of life and happiness, of futures and dreams. It leaves scars no one can see. But I know they are there.

There is no symbiotic relationship with leukemia. It doesn't share. It takes everything.

Maybe we become more introspective as we get older because we realize how short life can be. You learn that someday isn't coming; it's here. We have to appreciate what we have when we have it. You never know what the future holds or how you'll cope with a tragedy.

I remember the social worker at UC telling me years ago that parents whose children died after a long illness dealt with the death better than those who had a child die unexpectedly. I'm sure that's because death brings an end to the suffering when a particularly horrendous disease, such as leukemia is involved. But the loss is a loss, no matter how it happens.

I would experience the pain of losing a dear one unexpectedly when my mother was killed in an automobile accident in February 1983 caused by a man driving under the influence of drugs and alcohol. He veered into her lane with his big pickup truck and crashed into her small sedan.

She tried to swerve out of his path, but she couldn't get out of the way in time. My young nephew was in the car with her. Mom's evasive maneuver saved his life, but the trauma of the accident left him deeply shaken for years.

131

The driver was never punished because his girlfriend said she was driving, despite my nephew insisting otherwise. The man had a police record and she didn't. She ended up serving a few weekends in jail and paying a modest fine. The man saw my sister-in-law at a restaurant a few weeks after the trial and actually bragged to her how he got off scot-free.

My mother was a healthy sixty-seven, and I had anticipated she'd be around for several more years. Like Kari, I didn't get to tell her goodbye. Sometimes I'd forget that she was gone and reach for the phone to call her weeks after her death. She was a sweet, gentle lady and a great help to me in so many ways.

I will always miss her; and once again, I feel that I have been robbed of a loved one, because of unjust circumstances.

Joe and I are both retired now. I did end up continuing on in college and earned my teaching credential. It took me nine years to complete the five year course. I did most of it on a part-time basis, so I could be home with my girls as much as possible.

I taught for nineteen years and most of that time was spent in a self-contained classroom with third graders. They're usually eight years old when they begin the school year and nine by the time they're ready to move to the fourth grade. This is a wonderful age to work with. The kids are old enough to be pretty independent, but still young enough to believe the teacher might know a few things.

I will always be thankful I had the opportunity to spend time with these young children. I know I learned from them. Important lessons like, root for the underdog, share what you have when you see someone is doing without, and accept each other even if the other guy looks a little different than you or doesn't dress as well as everyone else.

Joe and I both truly enjoyed teaching and felt lucky to have chosen a profession that gave us such a sense of satisfaction. He received many distinguished awards during his thirty plus years of teaching, coaching, and counseling, including a prestigious grant to do graduate work at Oregon State University where he earned an advanced degree. He was also honored locally by being inducted into the Oroville Union District Hall of Fame in 2012.

He's enjoying his retirement by being active with golf and bowling, keeping a vegetable garden, going out to breakfast with a few buddies, and monthly luncheons with other retired teachers in our town. Speaking of town, Joe usually runs into one of his ex students when he's out. These people always have positive things to say about the time they spent in his classroom.

I tend to be more sedentary than Joe. I like to read, solve crossword puzzles, and work jigsaw puzzles. But my real passion is writing. I guess you could say I have a fascination with the written word. I've kept a daily diary since I was fourteen years old. I also enjoy writing poetry and I've had five romance suspense novels published.

Although Joe and I like different activities, we do share our interest in traveling, especially taking cruises. We took our first cruise in 1982 to celebrate our twenty-fifth wedding anniversary and have been hooked ever since. Hawaii is one of our favorite spots, but we've also spent time going to many other places over the years. I like to write about some of them in my books.

But I know I don't have to leave home to find happiness. I've learned contentment and beauty can come in unexpected ways like the morning after Michelle was married. I went into her bedroom still trying to take in the fact that my little girl was all grown up now.

Sunlight was streaming into the window and shining through the cutout appliqués on the train of her wedding dress. The sequins dotted the walls and ceiling with dozens of tiny rainbows.

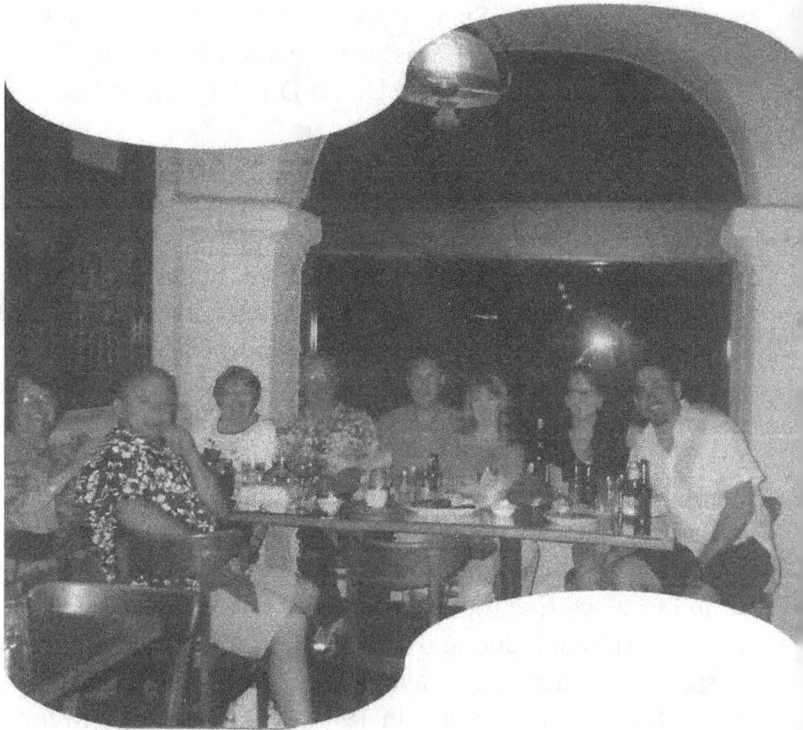

Our Grown-up Family: Our daughters with their husbands

I already mentioned that I like fall and the gorgeous colors of autumn. I also enjoy sunsets. That's what I would paint if I had the talent. I recall one particular evening when I was driving. The sun was just dipping below the horizon as I came around the bend in the road. The sky and the surroundings had suddenly turned to a beautiful shade of gold. What a breathtaking sight.

We haven't had the worry of Kari's illness hovering over us any longer, but life hasn't been without some stressful times since her death. I already wrote about losing my mother in such a violent way. Joe had a couple of serious issues with his health, including a tumor in his colon in 1993 and a blood clot on his brain in 1998.

The tumor incident made itself known by a lot of rectal bleeding late one night. Joe had just arrived home from a business teachers' conference and began to complain of stomach cramps. He ended up collapsing in the bathroom. I was able to get him to the hospital quicker than an ambulance because we live so close.

Walking into that emergency room wasn't easy. It brought back memories of our times with Kari. A pall of depression seems to hover over these places. Is it any wonder when you consider why people are there? We're not exactly talking Disneyland.

I'd heard unsettling stories of how people sometimes had to wait hours to be seen by a physician in our local hospital emergency room. I hurried to the check in window and told the woman how Joe had been passing quite a bit of blood. What a relief it was when she had me immediately lead him out of the waiting area and into an examining room. We were also fortunate to have a doctor come to exam him right away.

Joe ended up being admitted to the hospital. I stayed with him until he insisted I go home. It was after midnight by then. I always think emergencies seem much worse at night. I walked into our empty house and undressed for bed, but I didn't sleep. That old feeling of helplessness made a poor bed partner.

Joe was in the hospital for three days undergoing different tests before he was finally diagnosed with the tumor. He had to have surgery to remove the unwanted mass; thankfully he came through the operation fine. Even more good news was the fact that the tumor was benign. What a relief. It hadn't been a very pleasant experience, but it ended up being okay.

It's easier to suffer the scratch of a kitten than the claw from a lion.

We were in Missouri in the summer of 1998 for a family reunion, when Joe had the blood clot on his brain. It was very hot, and the humidity was brutal. He'd been swimming in the motel pool and came back to our room feeling nauseated and clammy. He also had a terrible headache and was a little disoriented. I thought he might be suffering from heatstroke.

One of my cousin's is a nurse and suggested we pack ice around his body. My brothers helped me, and Joe felt well enough by that evening to go out to dinner. But he woke up in the morning with another headache and spent most of the day in bed.

Our trip home turned out to be a nightmare in travel. The first flight left two hours late. Our connecting flight was delayed because lightning had hit the control tower, shutting down the airport. We had to sit in the plane on the runway for another two hours. By the time we finally landed in California it was the early hours of the morning, and we still had over an hour drive to Oroville.

I took Joe to our doctor that afternoon. He was examined and had some blood work done. It was suggested that he might be suffering from the flu. We were told to return in a couple of days for the results. Joe continued to suffer from the headaches. I didn't know what our doctor planned to do, but when I told him that things had not improved he ordered a CAT scan.

The technician came to us and said he knew what the problem was. The image clearly showed a blood clot. Our doctor sent us to the hospital in Chico a half hour away where a neurosurgeon was waiting to examine Joe. He told us he knew it was scary, but he wanted to give the clot a chance to dissolve on its own, so I brought Joe home after only one night.

He suffered through two days of nausea and vomiting. The headaches got worse. One of the things we were supposed to watch for was numbness. When I called to tell the surgeon Joe's hand had gone numb, surgery was scheduled for that day.

Two hours and twenty minutes later my family and I received the wonderful news that the surgery went well and Joe came through just fine. Whew! If you have to have a health crisis, it sure is nice when it's something that a doctor can fix. Nobody knows that better than I do.

I think I surprised the surgeon when I gave him a big hug, but I just couldn't help myself. By the way, he is one very fine doctor with an excellent reputation in his field. Little did I know at the time that our paths would cross again in the years to come when he ended up doing surgery on my back. I call him Dr. Miracle.

Oh, and I snuck in another hug then, too!

Chapter Eleven

We have had some good events going on in our lives, too. Joe and I both agree that one of the best things to happen for us in the last several years is becoming grandparents. Michelle and our son-in-law Rath gave us our first grandchild, a healthy baby boy named Rath, Jr born in April 1994. He was born in the Chico hospital. I felt a huge rush of love when I walked into the room and saw Michelle holding our new grandson.

I was still working at the time, and my principal knew how excited I was. She put the birth announcement in the school's weekly newsletter. Of course, I had to have his picture on my desk. I even had Michelle bring him to school one day to show off my handsome grandbaby. Incidentally, after having two blondes and two brunettes, I finally got my redhead in Rath, Jr.

He has matured into a fine young man that anyone would be proud to have in their family. He's twenty now, and attends college. He enjoys playing and coaching baseball just like his Grandpa Joe. He's an excellent student and a genuinely caring individual. I have no doubt that Rath will be a success at whatever he chooses to do.

I was also working when Joe and I became grandparents for the second time. We had a little granddaughter this time. Emily arrived in November 1996 to Kathy and our son-in-law Dave. They don't live in Oroville, and we weren't present at her birth. But, we went to see her soon afterward. What a beautiful, healthy baby she was with dark hair and eyes. Naturally, her picture went on my desk right next to Rath's.

Emily is eighteen and in high school now. She's quite the artist and enjoys playing water polo. She's also an amazing cook. You can't believe the fantastic recipes she creates. I'm sure she could easily make her mark in the culinary world if she decides to pursue that field.

Joe and I prayed for healthy grandchildren. We didn't want our daughters having to experience any heartache like we'd gone through. It really is a miracle of nature when you think about all the different parts that make up a healthy human being. We all know there aren't any guarantees that the baby will turn out perfect when a woman becomes pregnant. But we can hope.

My parents didn't have any idea that I would end up almost dying in infancy. I didn't expect Kathy to be born with a cleft lip, or that Kari would be diagnosed with leukemia. Was it so much to ask that this generation in my family would be spared more of this kind of sorrow?

We had two healthy grandchildren. So far so good, but it's like drawing straws. Sometimes someone comes up with the short one.

Our third grandchild, a little girl born to Michelle and Rath arrived in July 1998. She came a few weeks early and ended up being born on my mother's birthday. Was that a good omen? I guess it would depend on how you look at things.

I'm sure most people can relate to that instant clutch of fear you get when the telephone rings at night, jarring you awake. Joe took the call. It was Rath telling us that Michelle had just given birth to a little girl. He said they were working on the baby, and he would call us back later.

Working on her? What did that mean? I told Joe something must be wrong. Needless to say, we did not go back to sleep. How could we when our minds were so filled with apprehension?

Our son-in-law called again a few hours later. I listened while he described the baby's condition. I heard the distress in his voice and wondered why another misfortune had been thrust upon our family once again. Did we have some kind of target on our backs?

I hung up and immediately left for the hospital in Chico. Joe couldn't go with me because he was still recovering from his brain surgery just three weeks prior in the same hospital where our Michelle had now given birth to her little girl. I remembered going here after she had her son and how great it was walking into her room and seeing her holding her baby with our son-in-law standing so proudly by her bed.

I stepped out of the elevator and hurried down the hall, passing laughing and smiling people carrying brightly colored balloons, gift bags, and stuffed animals as I looked for Michelle's room. Whatever tears they were shedding were tears of joy. I wish I could say the same, but I didn't want to give into the luxury of releasing my sorrow, because I wanted to be strong for Rath and Michelle.

I steeled myself not to cry and entered her room. All I could think to do was to give them each a hug and tell them how sorry I was. I had a sudden sense of déjà vu thinking back to that night so long ago when my parents tried to comfort me after I'd learned about Kari's diagnosis. I guess we all have the urge to protect our children from hurt even when they're adults.

The baby wasn't in the room and I wondered if she was already gone. Rath had explained to me on the phone that she would have to be taken to Sacramento to a larger hospital because the Chico hospital wasn't equipped to take care of infants born with serious complications.

The door opened a short time later, and a man and a woman came into the room. The man was pushing what I thought of as a traveling incubator. He wheeled it over close to Michelle's bed. I peeked in through the glass and got my first glimpse of my new grandchild. She was drawn up into a tight little ball with her feet tucked under her tiny rump.

Her eyes were closed in sleep. She had long eyelashes and dark hair like her daddy's. I reached inside and for a few seconds had the opportunity to stroke her soft, velvety skin. I felt my heart swell with instant love and compassion.

The woman introduced herself as the nurse who would be traveling with the baby and the man as the ambulance driver. After she finished explaining some things about the baby and transporting her, she asked Michelle if the baby had a name yet. I wondered myself because I didn't know what names she and Rath had picked out.

Michelle nodded.

"Kari Elizabeth," she said.

I very nearly did cry then just hearing her say those two very special names. We had another Kari to love. Elizabeth was my mother's name. I hoped Mom would be looking out for this special baby. My birthday is two days after my mother's, and we used to celebrate together whenever we could. I missed doing that. Now I had the chance to share my birthday with my new granddaughter. It was certainly something to look forward to.

Michelle and Rath were given a few more minutes with their baby before she had to be taken away. He left for the hospital in Sacramento soon after. The doctor released Michelle, and I drove her home. I wanted so much to say something to comfort her, but I felt very inadequate.

This was my daughter, and she'd just been dealt a heartbreaking blow. Her birth had brought me such happiness and she should have been experiencing the same joy with her own little girl.

Instead, they were facing an unknown future.

I stayed with Michelle until that evening. She spent some of that time in her bedroom alone. She is a very composed person and isn't one to openly show her feelings. I did my best to deal with the phone calls and visitors who came to express their concern.

As I drove home that night I prayed that God would help my granddaughter and give Rath and Michelle the strength to deal with whatever was going to happen. I couldn't hold back my tears any longer. At first I didn't realize I was crying until my sobs broke the silence in the car. I don't like to cry, but I couldn't help it. I also wanted to be in better control before I went into the house because I didn't want to upset Joe. He was already dealing with enough anxiety.

Kari Elizabeth was eventually diagnosed with arthrogryposis. The condition affects her extremities and restricts her range of motion. But she has made extraordinary progress considering all she's had to overcome. Many things are a struggle for her, but she doesn't give up. Kari can't bend her fingers, but she has figured out a way to hold the needle to crochet. She likes to make dolls and created what she calls my *Kari doll* for my birthday this year. She made the doll with brown hair and a red dress. I have the little doll sitting on my bed. It's a sweet reminder of the two special Karis in my life.

I've written a little more about this grandchild because her indomitable spirit reminds me of my own Kari.

Remember how I said I learned a lot from my students? Well, anyone could learn a lesson from my granddaughter's grit and perseverance. She is a role model to many and has received recognition from her schools and our county for the inspiration she instills in others.

Kari is sixteen now and attends the same high school where her big brother and both parents went. It also happens to be the school where Joe taught for over thirty years. You can bet he would love to be a teacher now and have the opportunity to see his grandchildren there.

1998 ended up being a pretty rough year for the family. We had some other concerns besides what happened with Kari. I had two surgeries in January. They were elective, but I had some complications and had to return to the hospital. It took me a lot longer than I had originally anticipated to recover. Luckily, Joe was in good health at the time and able to take care of me until I got my strength back.

My father's health began to deteriorate noticeably that year. He was still living in his little apartment, but was showing signs of ever increasing mental confusion. He could no longer drive and had become quite dependent on us. He called Joe one day and was frantic because he could no longer understand how to take care of paying his bills.

Joe not only took over that responsibility, he was also very good about checking on Dad almost every day. One of the things he did was play a few games of cribbage with my father at each visit. My Dad had always loved the game, so I was happy that this was something he could still enjoy.

It was difficult for me seeing this once strong-willed man be so vulnerable. But he still had enough pride to not always ask for our help. One incident was when he was having trouble with his gout. It wasn't very long after Joe had his head surgery, and neither of us had been to see Dad in a while. I called him every day, and he finally told me he hadn't eaten in a couple of days because his foot hurt too much to walk or stand.

I knew he didn't want to tell me because of our situation, but I felt terrible that he'd been suffering. I cooked him enough food for a couple of days and went to see him. I stayed until he ate. I would have spent more time with him, but I was afraid to leave Joe on his own for too long.

Dad continued to live in his apartment, but he got to the point where he wasn't doing much of anything for himself. I was taking care of his laundry, grocery shopping, and preparing some of his meals. I tried having someone come in to cook for him a few days a week, but it upset him to have strangers in his home.

Aunt June was trying to help us by doing things for Dad. He was her big brother and they were very close. But she had to stop when she was diagnosed with a malignant brain tumor that year. Sadly, she died in 1999 while she was at her daughter's in Kentucky.

Dad suddenly started losing a lot of weight and became very pale toward the end of 1998. I noticed that he didn't seem to have much of an appetite. We took him to the doctor and some blood tests were ordered. It turned out that he was very anemic. Joe or I took him for weekly iron shots. That all stopped when one day the doctor called me into his office and said he was sorry to tell me, but my father had leukemia.

I couldn't believe it! That miserable disease had struck our family once again.

Dad passed away at home in December of 1998 nine days shy of his eighty-sixth birthday. I'm happy to say that most of the family was able to be with him before he took to his bed.

I remember him saying he was glad his life was drawing to the end. He was the oldest of seven children and always felt he was responsible for taking care of everyone. He lived fifteen years after Mom died. The last thing he said was how much he wanted to be with her again.

It's difficult to live with months of constant stress. It eventually begins to take a toll on your mind and body. Ask any soldier deployed in a war zone. Most of this time I'd been doing my best trying to stay composed, but 1998 just seemed to drag on with one crisis after another.

I felt bad that I hadn't been able to go to church as much as I wanted to. But one Sunday in September, a couple of months after Joe's head surgery I was finally on my way to mass. I was in the car and realized I was going to be late.

I'm not in the habit of speeding, but I figured this was one time where I needed to get going. Down went my foot on the accelerator and on went the flashing lights on the policeman's patrol car that I unfortunately hadn't noticed. I pulled over and tried to explain to the officer my situation at home and how I was trying to get to church after missing for several weeks. I was very upset and I know I showed it.

He asked if I wanted him to call someone locally.

Who did he have in mind? Michelle, who was dealing with Kari's fragile health? Joe, who was recovering from brain surgery? Or perhaps my dad, who was suffering from dementia?

I told him no. He handed me a ticket and told me to have a nice day. Really?

I didn't make it to church. I turned around and drove home. I went upstairs and cried my eyes out. I simply could not stop. I suppose all the months of anxiety had finally opened the floodgates. I'd heard a good cry is helpful. All it did was give me a pounding headache.

Some people told us that God only gives you what you can fit on your plate. He must have thought we were carrying around a huge platter considering everything that happened to us in 1998. Things got so bad that our friends started sending us cards and letters of encouragement as one misfortune after another continued to unfold.

But as they say, whoever "they" are . . . life goes on.

And indeed, life does go on. Our fourth grandchild was born to Rath and Michelle in February 2001. They named him Daxton. His middle name is Joseph after his grandpa. It's kind of a change for Joe having grandsons after fathering four girls.

Dax is a handsome fourteen-year-old with blonde hair. He was diagnosed with autism a few years ago. He attends the same middle school where his parents went and was recently named Student of the Month.

Joe and I thought we were done having grandchildren when we had a wonderful surprise a couple of years ago.

Erica and our son-in-law Kyle presented us with our youngest grandchild in May 2012. He's an adorable blonde, blue eyed little boy named Axel. Joe and I are getting a big kick out of watching him grow and seeing how his personality is developing.

I just hope we can be around to continue enjoying our grandchildren. I especially hope we aren't going to have anymore catastrophic events happening to our family.

Robert Louis Stevenson wrote the following:

We must accept life for what it actually is – a challenge to our very essence and quality without which we should never know of what stuff we are made, or grow to our full stature.

I think Joe and I have had enough of trying to prove '*what stuff we are made of.*' We'd just like to look forward to a nice, quiet old age.

But God forbid, if something else really bad does happen again, I can only pray that the Almighty will give us the strength and courage to endure it.

Epilogue

Some people will probably wonder why I wrote this story and bring up all the sadness again. I wanted to give an honest account of the kinds of difficulties a person might have to deal with in a long term illness like Kari's. I had people say to me after Kari died that they didn't realize what we were going through, and they would have done more for us if they had known how bad things were. But mostly we were lucky that our family and friends were there for us.

If you know of someone who is experiencing hard times for whatever reason, ask if there's anything you can do to help. Sometimes people forget about you after their initial concern. Don't take good fortune for granted. A so-called perfect life can be taken away very quickly. The hand you offer in support today may end up being the hand you reach out for help tomorrow.

I know I've written about a lot of unpleasant things that have happened in my family. But let's face it, the longer we live the more we're going to be exposed to ugly things. Ill fortune eventually breathes its bad breath on us all. I realize there are others who have had awful things happen to them too, but it's all relative.

This actually isn't the first time I wrote about my Kari. Joe and I self published a book a few years ago mostly for family and friends. Now I wanted to tell how our grandchildren are doing and add that we had our little Axel since I wrote the last story. Another reason for writing it was to help people better understand what happens to a family after going through a tragedy like we did with Kari. I can't speak for others, but I felt I could give some insight into how we're faring now.

I especially wanted to pay tribute to Kari and tell the world how bravely she fought to stay alive against terrible odds. It's important to me that people know Kari did exist; and how much she touched our lives, and the lives of others, with what little time she was allotted on this earth.

I didn't keep any of the money from the sales of the other book. I donated it all to an organization that helps families in our area with children suffering from leukemia, and I'd do it again. I was told sometimes these families need money for gas, groceries, or even buying Christmas gifts for their children. It's the least I can do when my child gave her life.

Several years after Kari's death, I told my then priest about the dream I had of seeing her in a coffin. He came to Oroville after she died, so I had to explain what had happened to her. He thought I was fortunate to have the forewarning. I don't agree. If anything, I was frightened that my horrible nightmare had come true.

Maybe someone else out there has had a terrible nightmare that came true like mine did and they're wondering if they are the only one. Or perhaps God spoke to them, too. Well now they know they're not alone. I don't have dreams about Kari now. I let my imagination do the envisioning. I like to picture her running and playing with Cuddles, or being with her grandparents. Most of all I want her to be well and happy, the way she deserves to be.

A man once told me that when you die, it's the end of everything. He insisted there isn't anything waiting for us but darkness. I don't want to believe that we end up in a black abyss. I'd rather think that Kari has crossed a bridge carrying her away from the misery and pain she had to endure. I hope she has found her own little piece of heaven, just as she told me she would.

Whenever she had trouble pronouncing a new word, or trying to master a new skill, she would say, "I'm just a little child."

Yes, she was a little child with a terrible burden that had been thrust upon her. It was a journey she should never have been forced to make. We received a tremendous outpouring of sympathy after Kari passed away, including many cards and flowers. One of the plants we received still flourishes in our house. We call it our Kari plant.

I feel certain Kari would have done a lot more good in the world if she'd been given the chance. Her doctors told us she did contribute valuable information to the medical field in their search for a cure for leukemia. But sad to say there's still so much to learn.

According to the Leukemia and Lymphoma Society, the leukemia rate for children and adolescents younger than 15 years in the United States has declined by 80 per cent in 1969-2010. But despite the decline, leukemia causes more deaths than any other cancer among children, adolescents, and young adults under age twenty.

Remember me mentioning the little girl who was the other *"old-timer"* with Kari at the clinic? Her father happened to be in Oroville visiting friends several years later. He recalled that we lived here and looked our number up in the phonebook. We would have liked to see him, but we weren't home. He left his number and I called him back.

It was like stepping back in time talking to him. We shared our memories. It was bittersweet, but it allowed us a chance to talk about our little girls. You never forget what it's like to have special children like them in your life. I was sorry to learn that his lovely wife had died a few years ago of breast cancer.

I attend St. Paul's Episcopal Church in Oroville regularly now; and when I do miss going, I can forgive myself. I want to trust that God will support me in my times of need. One of my favorite verses is, *Footprints.* I'm sure there are many people who can identify with that message:

God did not leave the person in their hour of need. He carried them. That's why there is only one set of footprints in the sand.

Joe still struggles with his belief in God because he cannot understand why bad things should happen to innocent children. We used to go to the cemetery and put flowers on Kari's grave to mark the date of her death. But we finally stopped. It's Joe's birthday, and better that we celebrate that.

It's not easy letting go of someone you love. But time gradually does help you wean yourself away from some of the sadness. A big part of who I am is bound up in my motherhood. Whenever anyone asks me how many children I have, I tell them three, but my heart says four.

I still see the woman now and then whose baby girl had to have heart surgery. The operation was a success, but tragically the girl died in an automobile accident when she was a teenager.

It's easy to feel smug when everything is going well in your life. Only a pessimist would sit around waiting for something bad to happen. I don't do that, but I am cautious in what I take for granted. We are very sad that we couldn't have Kari with us longer and that so much of her life had been filled with such suffering. But we will always be thankful that we had the opportunity to know this wonderful, wonderful child. That is where the true blessing lies.

Kari did tell me her time with us was limited in her words.

"Jesus needs me more," she said.

Obviously, He did.

About the Author

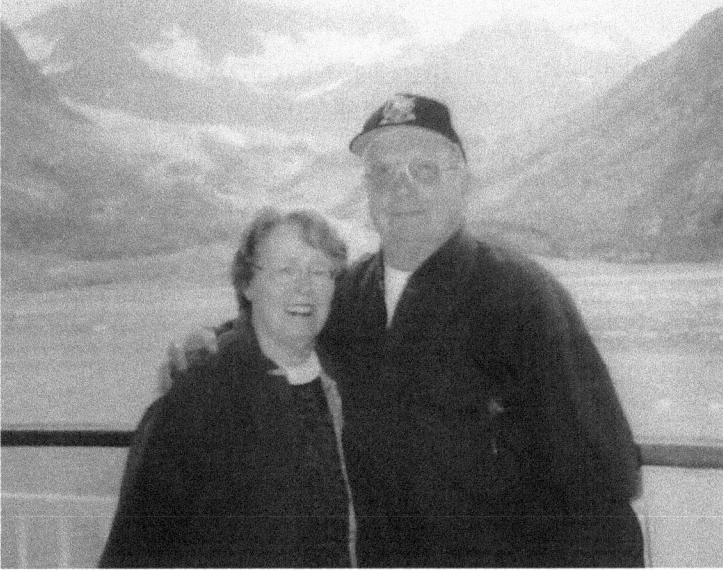

Claire & Joe ~ Cruising in Alaska

Olivia Claire High and husband, Joe have decided that their favorite type of vacation is to take a week-long, or preferably longer, cruise where Claire mixes sunshine and relaxation with gathering new material for her next romantic suspense novel. A prolific writer, she now has five published books and at least one in the hopper just waiting for her publisher.

Claire High is a former elementary school teacher, mother and grandmother. In addition to traveling, she also enjoys reading, writing novels and working puzzles. She and Joe live in Oroville, California where she is active with Curves exercise groups, her book club, and promoting her growing list of books.

Other Books by Olivia Claire High

Available at: www.firesidepubs.com or Kindle / Nook
& www.amazon.com

Other Books Published by Fireside Publications